NURSING AND RETIREMENT HOME ADMINISTRATION

NURSING AND

THE IOWA STATE UNIVERSITY PRESS

RETIREMENT HOME ADMINISTRATION

Edited By

H. Lee Jacobs, Ph.D.

and

Woodrow W. Morris, Ph.D.

The Institute of Gerontology
The University of Iowa, Iowa City, Iowa

AMES, IOWA, U.S.A.

This book was produced in cooperation with
the Iowa State Department of Health,
Iowa Nursing Home Association, and
the American Nursing Home Association.

First edition, 1966
Second Printing, 1966

Library of Congress Catalog Card Number: 66–12840

Foreword

> ***He who is with himself dissatisfied,***
> ***Though all the world find satisfaction in him,***
> ***Is like a rainbow-coloured bird gone blind,***
> ***That gives delight it shares not.***
>
> **—Thomas Hardy**

For the past three years groups of "dissatisfied" nursing and retirement home administrators have made their respective ways to the campus of the University of Iowa to participate in what was, in a sense, a series of experimental courses in nursing and retirement home administration. We are grateful to these people —over one hundrd of them—who came here from all parts of the state for about two days of each of five weeks to participate in a learning process designed eventually to help each of them in a process of self-improvement. To them this volume is dedicated.

As will be seen from the Table of Contents, this book is the work of many hands. So many hands, in fact, that not all the contributions made in the actual series of courses could possibly be included. We are most appreciative of the singular contributions of all these teachers, their willingness to help, and their patience in preparing copy and reading and rereading it.

While we hope this book will be regarded as a useful basic textbook for other courses in this field of educational endeavor, it is also our fond hope that individual administrators will find it useful as a reference in their own libraries or offices.

In any case it is with understandable pride, I believe, that we offer this volume as another evidence of the partial fulfillment of the purpose of the Institute of Gerontology: to perform and stimulate research in the aging process; to develop, to encourage the development of, and to carry on educational programs in aging; and to respond to requests for service programs to individuals, institutions, and communities with respect to the general welfare and status of the older person.

I would be remiss indeed if I did not express our gratitude to the Iowa State Department of Health, Division of Chronic Diseases, through which financial assistance was sought and received from the Division of Chronic Diseases, United States Public Health Service. I want also to thank the advisory committee members who helped to develop the plans for the course which is the basis for the book. They and their affiliations follow:

J. Leonard Davies, Ph.D., Associate Professor, Director, Bureau of Instructional Services, Division of Extension and University Services, the University of Iowa

Gerhard Hartman, Ph.D., Superintendent, University Hospitals, and Professor and Director, Graduate Program in Hospital and Health Administration, the University of Iowa

Adeline M. Hoffman, Ph.D., Professor, Textiles and Clothing, Department of Home Economics, and Affiliate Member, Institute of Gerontology, the University of Iowa

Terry B. Jones, Director, Physical Therapy, Department of Physical Therapy, the University of Iowa

Walter W. Lane, Construction Engineer, Division of Hospital Services, Iowa State Department of Health

John E. Muthard, Ph.D., Professor and Rehabilitation Counseling Psychologist, College of Education, University of Iowa

Mrs. Christena Nelson, R.N., Past President, Iowa Nursing Home Association, and Associate Administrator, Nelson Nursing Home, Fairfield, Iowa

Margaret A. Ohlson, Ph.D., Professor of Internal Medicine, and Director, Nutrition, University Hospitals, the University of Iowa

Jack E. Penhollow, M.D., Director, Division of Gerontology and Chronic Diseases, Iowa State Department of Health

Felix W. Pickworth, Director, Division of Hospital Services, Iowa State Department of Health

Ralph J. Quackenbush, Executive Director, Iowa Nursing Home Association

Merlin A. Taber, Ph.D., Associate Professor, School of Social Work, the University of Illinois

Betty van der Smissen, Dr. Recreation, Associate Professor of Recreation, the Pennsylvania State University

Pearl Zemlicka, Assistant Professor, College of Nursing, the University of Iowa

WOODROW W. MORRIS, Ph.D.
Director, Institute of Gerontology
Associate Dean, College of Medicine

Preface

The acknowledgment and understanding of the need for nursing and retirement homes carries an early awareness of the requirements for their efficient and effective administration. Certainly without such an awareness, the original need will not be well met. These goals can be realized only through "trial and error" experience or from a foundation of tested information and knowledge to which informed experience can be added. The latter seems to be the more reasonable and desirable approach.

This manual, supplementing as it does the presentation and discussions in the classroom sessions, is designed to help furnish this foundation of information and knowledge. Each author has been chosen on the basis of his distinctive qualification to deal with his allotted subject. Their work bespeaks these qualifications. It remains the responsibility of the reader and participant, in reading and listening, to benefit from the experiences, mistakes, and repetitive efforts of others and of the past.

For full acknowledgment of the efforts being given in the presentation of this course and the publication of this manual, much credit is due not only to the authors and lecturers but also to the time, energy, and attention contributed by the many who, through their administrative efforts, have added much to the success of this course and manual on administration.

ARTHUR P. LONG, M.D., Dr.P.H.

Contributors

DELORES A. BALTZ, M.S.
Administrative Dietitian, University Hospitals, the University of Iowa

FLORENCE L. BALTZ, R.N.
Past President, American Nursing Home Association; and Administrator, Washington Nursing Center, Inc., Washington, Illinois

ALTON E. BARLOW
Past President, American Nursing Home Association; and Administrator of the Canton Nursing Home, Canton, Ohio

MARGIE S. DAVIS, R.N.
Secretary, American Nursing Home Association; and Co-Administrator of Davis Nursing Home, Denver, Colorado

LEON I. GINTZIG, Ph.D.
Professor and Assistant Coordinator, Program in Health Care Administration, George Washington University, Washington, D.C.

THEODORE E. HAWKINS
Past Regional Vice-President, American Nursing Home Association; and Administrator, Hawkins Convalescent Home, New Haven, Connecticut

ADELINE M. HOFFMAN, Ph.D.
Professor, Textiles and Clothing, Department of Home Economics; and Affiliate Member, Institute of Gerontology, the University of Iowa

HENRY A. HOLLE, M.D.
Executive Director, National Council for Accreditation of Nursing Homes, Chicago, Illinois

H. LEE JACOBS, Ph.D.
Assistant Professor, Institute of Gerontology, the University of Iowa

TERRY B. JONES, R.P.T.
Director, Physical Therapy, Department of Physical Therapy, the University of Iowa

JEROME KAPLAN
Executive Director, Mansfield Memorial Homes, Inc., Mansfield, Ohio; and Associate Editor, The Gerontologist

W. E. KYLE
Past President, Iowa Nursing Home Association; and Administrator, Woodlawn Convalescent Home, Waterloo, Iowa

WALTER W. LANE, B.S.
Construction Engineer, Division of Hospital Services, Iowa State Department of Health, Des Moines, Iowa

ARTHUR P. LONG, M.D., DR.P.H.
Commissioner, Iowa State Department of Health; and Clinical Professor of Preventive Medicine and Environmental Health, the University of Iowa

JANET R. MACLEAN, DR. RECREATION
Associate Professor of Recreation, Indiana University, Bloomington, Indiana

ISABEL MACRAE, R.N., M.A.
Instructor in Medical-Surgical Nursing, College of Nursing, the University of Iowa

ANNABELLE L. MARTENEY, M.S.
Administrative Dietitian, University Hospitals, the University of Iowa

WILLIAM S. MOELLER, M.D.
Assistant Professor of Psychiatry, the University of Iowa

WOODROW W. MORRIS, Ph.D.
Director, Institute of Gerontology; and Associate Dean, College of Medicine, the University of Iowa

GEORGE T. MUSTIN
Past President, American Nursing Home Association; and Director, Wychmere Nursing Center, Memphis, Tennessee

CHRISTENA NELSON, R.N.
Administrator, Nelson Nursing Home, Fairfield, Iowa; and Past President, Iowa Nursing Home Association

MARGARET A. OHLSON, Ph.D.
Professor, Internal Medicine, and Director, Nutrition, University Hospitals, the University of Iowa

WILLIAM D. PAUL, M.D.
Professor and Director, Rehabilitation Unit, College of Medicine, the University of Iowa

FELIX W. PICKWORTH, B.S.
Director, Division of Hospital Services, Iowa State Department of Health, Des Moines, Iowa

WILLA A. SINGER, B.S.
Administrative Dietitian, University Hospitals, the University of Iowa

ROBERT A. SUTTON, B.S.
Assistant Director in Charge of Food Service, Department of Nutrition, University Hospitals, the University of Iowa

SHELDON S. TOBIN, PH.D.
Assistant Professor, Committee on Human Development, University of Chicago

EMMETT J. VAUGHAN, PH.D.
Assistant Professor, General Business, the University of Iowa

MERTON B. WEINER
President, Iowa Nursing Home Association; and Administrator, Westwood Convalescent Home, Sioux City, Iowa

Contents

PART VIII. STANDARDS AND REINFORCEMENTS IN THE CARE OF THE ELDERLY

Introduction

H. LEE JACOBS, *Ph.D.*

Nineteen million persons in the United States are now 65 years of age or over, with more than eight hundred being added per day. But the fastest growing segment of the entire population, from the percentage standpoint, falls in the age range of 85 years and up. In the decade 1950–1960 the rate of increase among those of this age was 60.8 per cent, as compared with 35 per cent for those over 65 years, and 18.5 per cent for the general population. More than two and one-half million have passed their eightieth birthday, and it is estimated that by 1970 there will be slightly under four million men and women in the 80-and-above age group.

Thus the problem of chronic illness, which as all evidence indicates is centered on this portion of the population, will continue. This fact was emphasized in the findings of the 1963 Survey of the Aged, conducted by the Social Security Administration. This survey showed that whereas only about one out of fifty persons aged 65 to 72 was in a nonhospital facility during 1962, the rate increased to one out of fifteen for those aged 73 and over. Because of this situation, along with the skyrocketing cost for hospital care (now twice as much as ten years ago and more than four times that of twenty years ago), plus the additional fact of important changes in family living patterns, the demand for more and better care for the elderly in the nursing and retirement homes is likely to mount.

What facilities are available to meet this growing need? In 1961 nonhospital facilities in the United States and its possessions which were providing nursing and supportive services to chronically ill and aged persons totaled 23,000, or 2,000 less than those estimated in a Public Health Service Inventory in 1954. These include nursing and convalescent homes, homes for the aged, rest homes, personal care homes, and boarding homes for the elderly, as defined and classified by the various states. Despite a drop in total number of facilities, however, the actual resident capacity of these homes had reached 592,000 by 1961, or a 32 per cent increase over the 1954 total of 450,000 beds. Moreover, due to the discontinuance of many very small homes and the trend toward the building of larger facilities, the average size of these homes has steadily increased. Over the past decade the national average in proprietary homes has jumped from nineteen to thirty-two beds. Most new homes today range in size from about fifty beds to as high as 450. And, it should be remembered, proprietary nursing homes comprise about 85 per cent of the total of such homes.

A most hopeful trend in the nursing home field is to be seen in the fact that the total beds in skilled nursing homes nearly doubled between 1954 and 1961. In 1961 skilled nursing care was the primary function of 9,700 nonhospital facilities, or 42 per cent of the 23,000 nursing homes and related facilities in this country. Beds in these facilities (338,700) accounted for 57 per cent of the total beds in all kinds of nonhospital facilities for the chronically ill and aged. As of December 1965, Iowa accounted for 822 of these licensed homes, with 23,902 beds, or 3.5 per cent of all homes and about 5 per cent of all beds.

The type of care for the aged supplied by nonhospital facilities is indicated in Table 1.1. A glance at the four main types of care makes it clear that although a wide variety of services is needed, by far the greatest demand is for the kind of care which nursing homes are best equipped to provide. This is because the impact of chronic illness becomes much more severe with age. Thus, as this "geriatric load" grows, the importance of the well-equipped and soundly administered nursing home facility will expand accordingly.

Recent surveys have shown that about two-thirds of the residents in nursing homes are 75 years of age or older, with the average being about 80 years. Because of their greater longevity and the fact that many more women than men in the later years are widowed, two-thirds of all residents in nursing homes are women. This means that among

TABLE 1.1

NATIONAL ESTIMATES OF NURSING HOME AND RELATED FACILITIES, BY PRIMARY TYPE OF CARE PROVIDED, 1961

		Number of Beds	
	Facilities	Total	Skilled nursing
Primary type of care[1]			
Total	*23,000*	*592,800*	*362,200*
Skilled nursing care	*9,700*	*338,700*	*337,300*
Personal care, total	*11,100*	*207,100*	*21,500*
With skilled nursing	1,400	83,100	21,500
Without skilled nursing	9,700	124,000	0
Residential care, total	*2,200*	*47,000*	*3,400*
With skilled nursing	200	12,400	3,400
Without skilled nursing	2,000	34,600	0

[1] The type of care provided to a majority of the residents.

Source: U.S. Department of Health, Education and Welfare, Public Health Service, Division of Hospital and Medical Facilities. *1961 National Inventory of Nursing Homes and Related Facilities.*

the residents of nursing and other types of homes for the elderly, as in the population generally, the problems of the aged are increasingly the problems of aged women. What this may mean, so far as nursing and retirement home planning is concerned, has not been seriously assayed as yet.

While the general physical condition of nursing and retirement home residents has apparently improved in recent years because of the growing rehabilitative emphasis in training programs for administrators and other personnel, there still is room for substantial improvement. In many cases administrators and staffs could render more efficient service if they possessed more accurate information on the nature and extent of chronic illness in the aging population generally and among their elderly patients or guests in particular. For example, many of them are not aware that impairment from chronic diseases is about twice as great for those 65 years of age and over as for all ages; that it is more than seven times as great at 60 as at 25 years; 15 times as great at 80 years as at 25; and that, at the same time, scientific evidence indicates that chronic illness and other disabling conditions are not necessarily characteristic of "old age," as such.

On the basis of a 1957 report (Table 1.2) on characteristics of nursing home patients in a *13-State Study* (Public Health Service Publication, 503), it is estimated that two out of three patients in proprietary nursing homes are suffering from cardiovascular diseases. One-fourth are considered "senile" (an ambiguous word), with more than one-third having periods in which they are disoriented "part to most of the time."

TABLE 1.2

DIAGNOSIS FOR PATIENTS IN PROPRIETARY NURSING HOMES[1]

Diagnostic Category	All Diagnoses	Primary Diagnoses
	Per cent of patients	
Cardiovascular diseases	65.6	40.3
Heart disease	17.2	11.6
Hemiplegia (mainly from stroke)	16.3	15.2
Other circulatory diseases	32.0	13.5
Senility	25.6	17.0
Fractures	11.3	8.8
Paralyses (excluding hemiplegia) and degenerative diseases of central nervous system	5.8	4.9
Mental disorders	5.5	3.6
Neoplasms	4.5	3.3
All other	39.1	12.8
No diagnosis	2.2	2.2

[1] Included 38,557 patients in a 13-state area study, 1953–54.

Source: U.S. Department of Health, Education and Welfare. *Nursing Homes: Their Patients and Their Care.* PHS Publication, No. 503, 1957, p. 13. (Joint Project of Commission on Chronic Illness and Public Health Service.)

According to the findings of this study one-fifth of all nursing home patients are confined to bed all of the time, and up to one-third part or most of the time. About 11 per cent of all nursing home patients sustain fractures, in most cases fractures of the hip. Some 6 per cent suffer from paralyses (excluding hemiplegia) and degenerative diseases of the central nervous system. Up to 6 per cent are afflicted with mental disorders, some 5 per cent by neoplasms, and 39 per cent by other complications. Less than half can walk alone and over one-third are incontinent. More recent survey data from selected states and local communities reveal similar findings concerning chronic conditions among elderly patients.

In the nation generally, 53.3 per cent of nursing home patients are supported out of public funds. On the other hand, a 1964 report from Iowa shows that 64 per cent of the patients in older proprietary nursing homes are welfare patients, as compared with 38 per cent in recently constructed proprietary facilities. This situation poses a serious problem for administrators, since the higher the percentage of welfare patients the greater the financial handicap to a home in its attempt to measure up to recommended standards of patient care.

With patient care costs rising at the rate of 5 per cent per year and with the many other problems facing administrators of nursing and other types of homes for the elderly, three steps, on which a modest beginning has already been made, should be promoted with increased vigor, namely:

1. The provision of more and better training for administrators (the general characteristics of this training have been briefly treated in the body of this manual);

2. Increasing emphasis on education of the public as to the very important service which nursing homes and homes for the elderly are rendering in a growing number of communities throughout the country; and

3. Closer scrutiny by legislative bodies of the problems and needs of these increasingly vital facilities for the care of the chronically ill and aged.

The administrator's role in the care of the elderly, in both nursing and retirement homes, is being steadily enlarged and his public image enhanced. This is being brought about through improved educational offerings in his field, as illustrated by the three-year demonstration project out of which the materials for this publication grew, and the professional associations, both state and national, to which he belongs. It is hoped that this volume will contribute in many practical ways to the further development and functional effectiveness of many administrators.

Part One

CARING FOR ELDERLY RESIDENTS

Chapter 1

Understanding the Elderly

SHELDON S. TOBIN, *Ph.D.*

In several of the chapters in this manual, the focus is on developing proficiency as an administrator; that is, on the skills and knowledge relevant to the services offered to those in need of care. Here, we shall begin by switching roles and placing ourselves in the position of the patient, client, or resident. (The word "resident" is used throughout when discussing the aged institutionalized person.) We then shall turn to the process of adaptation; followed by a consideration of those elements which may facilitate the process.

NEW RESIDENT'S POINT OF VIEW

The feelings of the new resident can be summed up in two global terms: helpless and hopeless. Helplessness is a feeling of loss of control, that one cannot affect the outcome of his or her life, and that many of the decisions of everyday living have been given over to others. Hopelessness is the more serious feeling of despair. It is a pervasive feeling that there is no future in one's life and that life has lost its meaning.

In discussing the feelings of helplessness in the aged person, Dr. Alvin Goldfarb (an eminent psychoanalyst in the field of gerontology), has stressed the need of people of all ages to feel competent, to be able to master some aspect of the environment. In individual psychotherapy with the aged, Dr. Goldfarb selects meaningful tasks which the patient can successfully master and which, when mastered, raise the feeling of self-esteem and self-worth.

Important components of helplessness are anxiety and guilt. Anxiety is a consequence of loss of control and the new resident who has lost the capacity to control everyday events in his environment may experience a reduced ability to control or modulate his own behavior. It is natural when experiencing this reduced capacity in oneself to turn to others for assistance and help. In turning to others, however, one may experience even greater feelings of impotence; indeed many older people feel that control of their lives has been ceded to others and this often evokes the fear that these others may misuse their power. This complex matrix of fears and anxieties is increased by feelings of guilt and shame. That is, the resident may feel guilty in accepting nurture from others and also ashamed that he cannot accomplish for himself many of the simplest tasks he formerly took for granted as being in his range of proficiency.

Apprehensive, anxious, and possibly guilty and ashamed, the new resident may develop a suspicious attitude toward the home; others are blamed for any and all of life's problems. This paranoia of the old is different from that of the young. To the older resident it has the meaning: "If you really loved me and were offering me honest assistance and help, then you would make me physically healthier and happier." This irrational expectation is in large part a consequence of accepting a dependent relationship with the staff of a home. While this expectation may be irrational it may also be necessary because it makes the new resident seek out and respond to help from others. (Indeed this expectation may also be necessary for the staff as well as the resident.)

This magical expectation that the institution will meet all their needs is comparable to the relationship between doctor and patient. In the typical doctor-patient relationship, the patient may consciously be aware that the doctor has no miraculous cures but still the patient expects magical cures. This expectation, unconscious as it often is, forms the fertile soil for a relationship between them.

A colleague of mine was recently comparing the magical expectations of the new resident to that which occurs in marriage. An elderly gentleman in the audience, a spry and wise old resident of a home for the aged, quickly retorted: "You may be right, but whoever heard of entering a marriage without a bride." Thus, while a magical expectation may exist, the new resident is more conscious of the losses which have occurred and which of these losses cannot be replaced by even the best of homes.

Hopelessness should not be confused with helplessness. To be without hope suggests a state of despair, where life has no meaning, and the future holds no chance of gratification. Many aged persons may feel depressed which is to be expected when we consider the many real losses which have been experienced, but the despair of the aged is quite distinct from the mood state we label "depression." Despair, indeed, can occur at any age. This was illustrated in a recent article in *Time* magazine, which reported the case of an adolescent hemophiliac boy who began to bleed uncontrollably when his father died. Somehow he felt guilty about the death of his father, with whom he had a very close, affectionate relationship. In this state of despair, all the advantages of modern medicine could not stop the bleeding.

Shortly thereafter he went into a coma and in this comatose state began talking about his father's death. He then suddenly responded to the medication. On waking from the coma he talked about the dreamlike state he had just been in, and how he had arrived at the conclusion that he was not at fault for his father's death and that life had meaning despite his death. This dramatic story illustrates the role of hope in physical illness, a phenomenon which is clearly evident among many new residents in homes. Recent studies by Dr. Morton Lieberman of the Committee on Human Development at the University of Chicago suggest that death among residents during their first year in the home is not related to degree of physical illness, but rather to the lack of feelings of hope and faith in the future.

Lack of hope is probably related to the attitude that a nursing or retirement home is a place to die. Entering a home when one is old and has many physical ailments can readily evoke this attitude. Also, by the age at which most people apply for admission, they have lost spouse, friends, and oftentimes children.

Hopelessness may be related to feelings of family rejection. The expectation of older people in our society is that their children will offer emotional support, especially in times of need. As Dr. Ethel Shanas, also of the Committee on Human Development, has found in a national survey, this expectation is in terms of comfort and assurance rather than financial assistance. Independent of the realities that necessitate institutionalization, the new resident may feel that the emotional support of children has been withdrawn; that he is being cast aside or put out to pasture to die.

Generational differences between parent and child often make it difficult to arrive at a mutually comfortable arrangement between them. The parent may feel very strongly that to leave the children's home is an insult to them even though the parent would be more comfortable making other arrangements. In urban areas, it is often seen that people of foreign birth have expected their children to succeed, and indeed their children have succeeded and have now moved out to the suburbs. When their elderly parent goes to live with them, the parent usually is unhappy because his child has retained little from the old country. In rural areas there are similar conflicts. A person who has lived, worked, and reared his family on a farm may feel alienated from his children who have moved to the city and succeeded. Even where a good relationship exists between the elderly parent and child, conflicts are usually present.

Thus, in entering a home, the new resident has to confront these deeply experienced feelings of helplessness and hopelessness. In turn, the staff of the home has a difficult task in assisting the new resident in his adaptation to the home, which assistance necessitates understanding the resident through his internal framework.

INSTITUTIONALIZATION

The unfamiliarity of the surroundings in the home for the aged creates major difficulties for the older person who has many established routines. Indeed it is also very difficult for younger persons to have their routines disrupted by a change of living arrangements. The older person differs from a child, however, in that a child entering a home may find it a new and exciting world while the elderly resident desires a stable environment. A difference, however, which can be exploited to great advantage, is that the adult has had mastery experiences which have enabled him to meet the challenges of everyday living for many years.

Adaptation to a Home

In a new surrounding one cannot but expect some disorientation at the very beginning. Obviously, the more similar the institution is to the resident's previous living conditions the less will be the degree of disorientation. Thus, there is a need for a diversity of homes. Recently a home which was physically dilapidated was described to me by a colleague. This woman said she was surprised she felt so comfortable in this old and somewhat dusty home—until she realized that the residents seemed unusually cheerful. Fortunately, the administrator of this home screened her new residents very carefully, selecting only those who shared her easygoing attitude.

No matter how well the match between resident and institution, it is to be expected that the initial adaptation period is a traumatic one. It is traumatic because of the feelings of insecurity inherent in adapting to such a new and different physical and social milieu and in adjusting to feelings of helplessness and hopelessness. Dr. Jerome Grunes, a psychiatric consultant at the Drexel Home in Chicago, has labeled the symptoms seen during the initial adaptation to the home as the "First Month Syndrome." He anticipates that any new resident will deteriorate during the first month, but will most likely reintegrate at the end of this period. In fact, if, in his clinical judgment, a person does not undergo such a period he then diagnoses him as psychotically unresponsive to his environment and therefore unable to make an institutional adjustment. With elderly people it is not surprising that they deteriorate and show a "First Month Syndrome"; rather, it is surprising that they maintain the integration that they do. From a biological standpoint it is apparent that central nervous system deterioration begins early in life, and that a loss of brain cells begins in the fourth decade of life, the loss accelerating with age. The maintenance of functioning, however, exceeds the structural loss of cells. So, too, in coming out of a syndrome, which appears at first to be an irreversible senile state, the older person is able to reintegrate in spite of cortical deficit.

This process of adaptation is congruent with one's earlier experiences in that the manner of coping with the stressful environment relates to the life style of the person: for example, the flirtatious and coquettish woman of eighty who always has related to others as a young, attractive girl. Her earliest memory reflects this orientation. The memory is of standing in front of a classroom dressed in the prettiest of clothes, at age six, performing for her classmates while they respond with love and attention. Throughout her life this has been her pose; and, indeed, her expectation of others.

In the adaptation process the new resident will choose those from among the staff with whom he wishes to interact. This interaction usually takes the form of early family relationships—as it did with the coquette of eighty years who related to the director much as a favorite daughter to a benevolent father. The staff also takes part in this selection process, as was illustrated by a recent study.

Staff Relationships

When I asked the staff at Drexel Home to list the best and least adjusted residents I found that many chose residents as the best adjusted whom others chose as least adjusted. In discussing their choices the staff revealed that highly personal relationships are developed between themselves and individual residents. Residents with certain personality characteristics select specific staff members with whom to interact. Likewise, the staff members make their selections. It would seem essential, therefore, to have a staff composed of a wide range of personality types. That is, a staff which has members who like the rebellious resident, others who like the more withdrawn or depressed resident, others who like to mother the very ill, and others who like the outcast or misfit. The tendency to obtain a staff which reflects the attitudes and personality of the administration should be counterbalanced by this need for diversity of personality types.

The administrative hierarchy also influences the interactions of staff and resident. The working relationships between director and associate director, for example, is usually perceived, or felt, by the residents and this influences their interpersonal interactions. The new resident will usually learn the network of these staff relationships through the older residents with whom they tend to relate as siblings. This learning is part of the initial adaptation process in which the new resident is taught "who is who" and how to relate to the variety of authority figures.

In adapting to the institution the new resident attempts to maintain his integrity while learning the many rules necessary for maintaining an efficient home. The maintenance of feelings of personal integrity in institutional living often takes interesting forms. In adapting to jails, for example, it has been found that the prisoners who are psychologically the healthiest often are sent to solitary confinement. In jail, solitary confinement is very important to the healthier prisoners because prisoners have no privacy and all movements are extremely regimented. Also, in a home for the aged, the form that mental health may take may often be disagreeable to the administration. Fighting with the administration, as many older people do, may reflect their need for autonomy and the need for blaming others rather than blaming themselves. It is often difficult to blame oneself for insufficiencies, and it may be a very positive thing in the older person to externalize and to project the blame onto others. Also the combative resident is truly engaged in interaction and thus does have feelings of hope. On the other hand, it is the passive and depressed resident who offers no administrative problems who may lack hope.

MASTERY AND DEPENDENCY

In working with older people, we have two types of expectations. First, we wish to fulfill their needs for physical care and to be responded to for our concern. At the same time we wish to encourage their mastery and control of their world. That is, we paradoxically wish to encourage them to accept our care while we also wish that they act as mature, competent adults. It is difficult for many residents to accept the care we are offering; and oftentimes residents will seek to gratify their needs for dependency and closeness in ways we do not desire. One way, for example, is provocative sexual behavior which, more often than not, reflects a need to have physical contact, to get close to other people.

We should look at our own motives in caring for older people. In working with older people, one of the gratifications is the attachment they may develop for us and the sense of accomplishment if this attachment leads to increased comfort and increased competence (or rehabilitation if we use this word in its larger sense).

Increased competence for the older person obviously takes a different form than for younger persons. If we use an example from physical medicine, for the hemiplegic who is lying on his bed and is incontinent, bladder control represents the mastery or competence that he desires at the moment. For many older people, what is most meaningful is the ability to structure the day, and it is in this structuring of the day that feelings of gratification are met. We must not equate mastery and activity, however. Mastery often necessitates little activity and indeed is more a psychological than a physical entity. It is a feeling of control over some part of the environment. Residents often are afraid that their dependency needs will not be gratified if they allow themselves to be too competent. We will expect too much of them. Under this fear that dependency need satisfaction will be withdrawn, many residents prefer to act somewhat childish or incompetent.

This complex area of mastery and dependency needs further exploration. From our standpoint we wish neither to encourage regression of residents to an infantile level of care and feeding, nor to encourage their acting like young, active twenty-year-olds. We must, however, offer each resident a feeling of security while encouraging a feeling of competency in those areas which are most meaningful to him.

RELATING TO RELATIVES

Another very important area is that of the resident's relationship to his relatives and the relationship of the administration to these relatives. Handling the guilt and anxiety of relatives often takes more of administrators' time than the care of patients. Unless these guilt and anxiety feelings are handled properly they may be very disruptive to the resident and to the home. One way they can be handled is to facilitate the relatives' identification with the institution as a whole. Often, the institution can be a symbolic parent replacement to the adult child of a resident. The child of a patient who is undergoing deterioration may find it very comfortable to shift his feelings or love from his parent to the institution as a whole. He is able to then say to himself that if this home is taking good care of his parent, he then is fulfilling his responsibility. This certainly should be encouraged when relatives feel both guilty and angry at their parents. Visits from children can often be very upsetting; and certainly less visiting needs to be encouraged at times.

DEATH AND THE LIFE REVIEW

One area which is consistently not talked about is that of death. To younger people it is very difficult to understand how it is that many older residents are able to die with equanimity. It is also very difficult at times to understand how there is not more mourning over the death of a resident of a home. The latter phenomenon is not so unintelligible. Many have had the experience of one nurse at a home who was able to predict who was going to die. So, too, residents seem to be able to sense or predict who among them is preparing for his own death. It appears that before the moment of death, people do prepare by slowly withdrawing from those around them. The mourning period appears to begin at this time and is probably completed by the time of physiological death.

The person himself who faces death at a late age has to, in some way, reconcile himself with his maker. Recently, Dr. Robert Butler, a psychiatrist at the National Institute of Mental Health, has used the term "life review" to describe the reminiscence that older people undertake in their later years. Within this life review are many ruminations and thoughts about the earlier life, and if, while reviewing one's life, it is possible to accept oneself and to say that life has been meaningful and purposeful, then it is easier to face death with equanimity. In this life review, we find a need to view oneself from a stable position. This stable position is usually how one was when one was younger and not how one is now. At the same time it is important to be able to say that "I lived a life and that I had only one life to live, and that was the only way it could be." I think we could sum it up by the following: "Don't evaluate me as I am now, because I don't evaluate myself as that, but evaluate me as I have been and what I have contributed."

In this reevaluation of himself (when the individual is really able to understand himself) one sees very honest, straightforward answers to questions and to life. I asked an elderly man recently why he had not married, and he said very simply that he had always been attached to his mother. He continued to talk about competing with his brother and many other things. In a young person such a response is indicative of severe disturbance, but not so in the old. This man, however, is able to understand it and to integrate it into his life scheme. He may not like his life style and how he lived it, but he can integrate it and he does have some positive feelings about himself. Lastly, it is important to the older person to have some identification with the world around him, and some feeling that his progeny (or persons or organizations in which he has invested) live on worthily after him.

CONCLUSIONS

In understanding residents from their perspective, the administrator often finds that smooth institutional functioning is at odds with residents' desires. The astute administrator will recognize not only this incongruence when it exists but will assess his own responsibility in the matter also. Thus, when aware that aggressive behavior for a particular resident is a sign of health, he will not avoid the issue by overcontrolling nor will he be overly permissive (which could be disruptive to other residents). Compromises which necessitate great flexibility need to be made constantly. This flexibility, in turn, can be accomplished only by individualization of services. That is, by treating each resident as a separate individual. To accomplish this goal the staff must be trained to understand the typical problems of the aged person; the specific problems confronting the new resident; and the highly personal set of problems of each resident.

Chapter 2

How To Cope With Emotional Problems

WILLIAM S. MOELLER, *M.D.*

Recently a 64-year-old gentleman said to me, "If they can operate on my heart and tell me I have only a 25 per cent chance of surviving the operation, I will do it." He went on to explain how he would prefer taking this risk, in order to live a somewhat normal life, instead of being chronically disabled and in need of constant nursing and medical attention. I immediately began to think about why this person would take this chance and why he would be concerned about chronic disablement. He has always been an independent man and an exceedingly hard worker with grand and ramifying accomplishments. He still has a very active and engaging mind. He adheres to many of the Old Country value systems and has never wanted to be dependent upon anyone.

Supposing chronic hospitalization or the need for nursing home care occurred, would the people with whom he would be forced to live understand him? Would they look at him other than as an older man with a tired heart? Could they be aware of his concerns about foods, grooming habits, reading habits, bowel habits, and visiting habits? Even if they could avail themselves of this knowledge, could they treat him and relate to him, in view of these understandings? And even if these things could be done, how would they deal with the realization that he did not want to be there; that he resented the implications of his being there; and that he might resent the people about him? Could they appreciate his concerns and know what to do with his pessimistic attitudes, tearfulness, his lamentings of the past? Then I wondered if he were in a place for this type of care, would it be close by? Would I see him frequently? And how could I handle his attitude of not wanting to live with his children and be a "burden"? The questioning continued. But by this time I was not repeating the curious ruminations of an uninvolved, seeking mind, but reacting as a layman, as a psychiatrist, as a physician, as a son; for this man is my father and these questions are not answered.

But as I thought about these things I was reminded of some of the problems involved in coping with the emotional needs of "elderly" patients in nursing homes. Then I became angry, because, a short period before, a nursing home administrator had told a friend of mine he resented all those blankety-blank people coming in to tell him how to run his home. Eventually my resentment faded into curiosity as to the origins of his attitude. This man runs a good nursing home. To my knowledge he practices most of the things which I certainly advocate, except for one thing which I will discuss later.

Since seven years ago, when I first organized a series of workshops throughout the state for nursing home administrators, I have had the opportunity of talking to and becoming friends with many of these people. I have visited many homes. I have referred many patients. I have talked with many patients from nursing homes. I have visited in many of these facilities and talked with nursing home administrators in other states. I have read the various nursing home publications since 1954, and I can say that in the last ten years a revolution in the nursing home field has taken place.

The uneducated criticism of these facilities, prevalent in the past, is greatly diminished. Self-education and consultation programs on state, local, and community levels have abounded, and the true professionals in the field have continuously searched for useful ideas. In addition, there is a state-wide nursing home day once a year. Where these efforts on the part of administrators have not been sufficient, they have been augmented by the developing concept of community responsibility that abounds in all areas of medicine, especially in that of psychiatry.

A wholesale removal of patients from psychiatric institutions with placement in community nursing homes has occurred, but the greatest change of all has been the growing tendency for physicians and others to question what has been so characteristically accepted in the past, namely, that extreme dependency, morbidity, and mortality among older people are inevitable concomitants of advancing age. We are at long last aware that our erroneous notions about age have been responsible for much of the depression and confusion that exists in elderly patients. We are less likely than formerly to apply the term "senile brain changes" in our diagnoses.

MEDICAL ASSESSMENT AND TREATMENT

It is, of course, absolutely essential that the physical ailments, the diseases which ravage patients, have excellent medical assessment and treatment. Physicians generally are quite capable of diagnosing and prescribing treatment for these conditions. The experienced administrator is also apt to be aware of diabetes, chronic syphilis, arteriosclerosis, senility, depression, adjustment reactions to stress, loss of loved ones, and the like.

As I see it, training for the administrator in the efficient management of a nursing home includes some instruction in such matters as the correct use of tranquilizers, antidepressants, insulin, physical therapy techniques, how to prepare diets of various qualities and quantities, and adequate knowledge of fireproofing techniques. The administrator also needs training on how to educate the community concerning the needs of the elderly and what is involved in adequate patient care. Above all, it must be impressed upon him that he is providing care for people who have chronic ailments and who are often hopeless and dying, due in no small way to our society which has characteristically given little role to the elderly person and has tended to reject and isolate him.

What evidence do we have for programs calculated to involve the elderly as well as the young? Is it true that the average physician, seeing a bedridden, incontinent, confused patient sets the same therapeutic goals involving the restoration of this man into some working involvement in the community, or thinks of returning such a patient with a newly fractured hip to living in and caring for his or her own home? Indeed not! For he has long considered the phenomenon of arteriosclerosis and senility as end points, with irreversible physical disintegration. As administrators you should think about these things and bring yourselves to the realization that indeed the fundamental error we all make in trying to cope with the problems of the elderly and the elderly ill is that we approach them through treatment of their organ systems, with lack of awareness of their healthy parts, and that, moreover, we treat them with abounding pessimism. This pessimism accounts for the most serious emotional problems in nursing homes.

Now, lest it be charged that these strivings come from an ivory tower, let me cite some cases with evidence.

Patient Number One: This 66-year-old woman was referred by a nursing home and relatives, with a question about a rehabilitation program with goals of decreasing physical disability and increasing her motivation to participate in daily events. It was noted on admission to our hospital that this woman spoke only in whispers and her whispering was very difficult to understand. Most of her answers to questions consisted of nodding or shaking her head. Her hand was so unsteady that her handwriting was almost illegible. This patient had been confined to a nursing home for six years prior to admission. The administrator reported crying spells had been present for about five years; recently these had occurred once every two weeks. The patient had gradually lost her ability to speak over the past three or four years and had been spoon-fed over the last two years. What precipitated the psychiatric consultation was the statement the patient made to her son when he visited recently in the nursing home. Her son had been attempting to communicate with his mother in their accustomed fashion when his mother suddenly spoke out in a clear tone and said, "Can't something be done for me?" Prior to the patient's admission to the nursing home, she had had a left mid-thigh amputation of the lower extremity, presumably because of embolism. She had complained of phantom leg pain ever since. She had been given morphine and codeine for this pain by the local physician, and it had been reported that two years prior to admission her consumption of codeine tablets was as high as 200 tablets every two weeks. The local physician, recognizing the addiction to codeine, had apparently successfully withdrawn the medication prior to admission.

Her past history, outside of significant material related to the family that I will not go into, indicates the loss of one of her sons in an automobile accident, and, at about the same time, the mid-thigh amputation. After two years in a nursing home, her only daughter had moved far away, and from that time on the patient had lost her ability to speak. Before becoming ill, she was described as having been lively, talkative, optimistic, kind, and hard working. She had been in good health during her life until 1954 when she had a hysterectomy. During this operation she apparently had a cardiac arrest which necessitated cardiac massage. She apparently also had extensive embolizations after her hysterectomy. She became depressed after her son's death and soon suffered a cerebral vascular accident which has left her with a neurological deficit. Now involved in that particular year of losing her son, experiencing the depression, the stroke, and the amputation, she also had a kidney removed. Her past history also indicated cardiac disease and irregular pulse, mild hypertension, diffuse heart murmurs and heart fibrillation, pitting edema, amputation, muscular weakness in her right leg, coarse tremors of all of her extremities. During hospitalization extensive evaluations were made and the patient was seen by the Departments of Internal Medicine, Orthopedics, Ophthalmology, and Oral Surgery. As much was done to give attention to these complaint areas as humanly possible and several actions were taken. During hospitalization the patient's previous medication, which included Nembutal, Darvon, and Phenobarbitol, were gradually removed with the patient showing no withdrawal symptoms. She adjusted rapidly to the ward and did very well with the ward routine.

The therapeutic approach was initially of a supportive nature, but later on it was one of a more reeducative nature. She responded beautifully and at the time of her discharge she was able to carry on extensive conversations in normal tones. Her handwriting had become quite legible, her interests in general had returned, and her tearfulness had been eliminated. This was accomplished in a little over four months hospitalization. This patient's progress was of such a nature that she was now able to return to the home of her family. Over a year later she wrote while in Texas that she had also spent some time with her daughter in California. Her writing was quite legible and she indicated that she was doing well, that she was reading books, etc.

All of this improvement, I suggest to you, was premised on changes in attitude on the part of the nursing home administrator, the son, and the patient.

Patient Number Two: I refer here to a younger patient, but certainly one in whom an attitude of hopelessness was markedly present. This is the case of a 44-year-old man who had been at one of the state mental health facilities from 1945 to 1963, when he was transferred to our institution. This man had a diagnosis of chronic paranoid schizophrenia. After being in the state hospital for these eighteen years, he was transferred to our hospital at our request because we were interested in seeing what environmental change could do. This is in conjunction with our studies to see what can happen with a change in attitude toward people who have been in a state of hospitalization for many years. His history indicated illness had begun two years prior to his admission to the state hospital and had occurred following the death of his mother. Apparently, after her death, he had lost all self-confidence and was not able to make out in his farm work. He refused to clean himself and was considered a nuisance. It was therefore felt necessary to get him out of the community. After commitment to the state hospital he showed further regression.

In spite of this, the patient was able to make a generally satisfactory adjustment, although he did not talk much and was able to carry out only menial tasks. He was in our hospital four months. The essential therapy was that of milieu therapy in which the personnel attempted to form a close relationship with him. This had been successful and he seemed to respond and open up more with people who tended to spend considerable time with him. He formed fairly close relationships with the student nurses. His sister, who was very cooperative in working with the patient, made weekly visits, took him out for rides, and to her home for meals. She seemed to reestablish meaningful contacts with him. He seemed to enjoy these visits, looked forward to them, and participated in them. While in the hospital he was able to participate in games and other activities and demonstrated ability to perform uncomplicated tasks in lines of work. He was not treated with drugs, and was eventually transferred to a nursing home. He was taken on daily visits to the home and each time allowed to stay longer. When he became accustomed to the place, he was invited for dinner and then for weekends. Later he spent longer periods of time in his contemplated room. He began to like the home very much and was pleased with the eventual transfer. Follow-up contacts are being maintained, but this story is not yet completed. It will be absolutely essential here that the outside contacts be maintained; that the individual be involved in work tasks that are meaningful; and that close relationships continue to develop and flourish. However, these things cannot indeed be the end. In the months ahead further progress should be expected.

In the first patient's case we see that over a period of years a nursing home was able to break through to the patient and produce the needed motivation. While it took too long perhaps, when the motivation was discovered, the opportunity was seized upon and movement occurred. The second patient does not reflect the average patient in the nursing home. I well recognize that the bulk of individuals in a nursing home are over the age of eighty. Yet I know that many patients are transferred now (and will be in the future) from state hospitals. In the future they may be of younger ages. What I did not tell you about the second case was that a number of years earlier he had been precipitously transferred to a county home. He immediately ran away from this home, was exceedingly difficult to control, and was returned to the state institution, where he remained. The brief description I gave of the process of transfer from our hospital to the nursing home involved the point I now wish to make.

We knew that this patient was long prepared for this transfer to our institution, and we actively planned the gradual transfer to the nursing home. It has been long felt that patients going to state hospitals die early. This has often been thought due to the care they received, but it is becoming fairly well established that the problem lies simply in their going to the state hospital.

HANDLE EMOTIONAL PROBLEMS EARLY

To elaborate, I would first suggest that the emotional problems that are witnessed by you can best be handled early by prevention and amelioration. After the patients have become combative, exceedingly depressed, or exceedingly excited, you, uniformly, must resort to the use of drugs. I suggested in 1959 at the Seventh Annual Nursing Institute here that every nursing home administrator make an intensive, thorough study of each patient's past history and personal life, in order to obtain a keen comprehension of his likes, his needs, and his fears. I indicated this would have to be done through relatives, friends, doctors, and through personal interviews with the patient, if possible. I felt then and feel now that it is essential these things be done prior to the patient's entering the nursing home and that the patient be prepared for this event. I feel it is necessary that each patient have an opportunity to meet you and learn to like you prior to his coming into your home. Let him have an opportunity to understand the program you are setting for him and your individual interest in him and try to discourage the attitude that he is being forced to come here as a last resort. Establish, rather, that you want him to come and that he will want to come. These things cannot occur in a matter of an hour but should occur over a period of days or weeks. It is to be recognized that upon meeting you he will not accept you or your programs easily or rapidly. There may be a lot of negativism expressed through hostile projections, but this must be approached through acceptance without becoming upset yourselves.

The first great premise in preparing anyone for something he does not like is to hope that he will express his negative, hostile feelings, and, if outbursts in the future are to be prevented, these feelings must be expressed fully initially. It can be expected that after the negativism has been expressed, the fears and doubts verbalized, he will begin to ask questions and show interest and be amenable to suggestion. It is this initial period that is of the greatest importance. This will set the stage for the next weeks, months, and perhaps years. The significance of these observations has been highlighted dramatically by the study reported in 1963 by Doctor Aldrich of the University of Chicago. He observes initially in his study that relocation of elderly people is done with risk, but that many factors are involved in high death rates. However, the closing of the Chicago Home for Incurables provided him and his associates with an opportunity to study aged inpatients who were relocated from one institution to another. This move was not related to the state of health, or family relationships, but was solely an administrative necessity. The movement was quite precipitous for fifty-seven patients; the rest of the patients in the study had some opportunity for preparation; however, all knew they were going to better physical surroundings. I cannot go into all of the statistics and details of investigation in this study but rather wish to give you its conclusions.

This study involved 233 patients. They were followed for a two-year period after the announcement of the closing of the home. Fifty-one patients died before leaving the institution. For the 182 who were relocated, the overall death rate one year later was 32 per cent. Results of this study indicated that when disabled persons, particularly the elderly, are transferred from one institution to another, for reasons which have nothing to do with their health or their family's attitude, there is a marked increase in the death rate, especially in the first three months following relocation.

Although the mere expectation of relocation was associated with an increase in the death rate, the increase was not statistically significant. The helpless and psychotic or near psychotic patients were the ones with the highest death rate in the first year after relocation. While this study cannot be considered absolute in its determinations, it was felt that the patients' psychological adjustment to the institutional life before the anticipation of relocation and the emotional response to actual relocation were significant in determining survival. It has been concluded that communication with the psychotic or near psychotic or helpless was quite poor. Adequate psychological preparation for the transfer did not occur. This study reflects the problems involved in transferring patients from institutions to nursing homes and may not be analogous to all your patients' situations. It does, however, highlight the important significance of the psychological involvements in the production of depression, also, motivation and death. I myself accept this as further corroboration that preparation in the sense of encouragement of expression of the patient's negative feelings and the development of a philosophical attitude, should be accomplished whenever possible. This will do much for the prevention of emotional problems in nursing homes. As administrators you should also recognize how important it is that patients develop confidence in you, like you, and be able to communicate with you.

MOTIVATIONAL TECHNIQUES

An additional gimmick in trying to prepare patients for the home you direct might be the involvement of a patient or two from the home with a prospective patient. Alcoholics have long since found themselves greatly influenced by other alcoholics through the AA, and teenagers communicate better with each other. I am sure each of you could cite many examples to corroborate the theory that patients can accept things from one another, oftentimes more readily than they can from the authority figure. Be sure, of course, to take along one of your most satisfied residents.

Now, I know that many homes are using occupational therapy, recreational therapy, TV, visitor programs, churches, clubs, and organizations. There was a time when most nursing home administrators were reluctant to make use of such facilities and of other people outside their homes. This was probably a natural reaction to feelings that they were being paid to do the job and therefore must do it alone. Also, their experience with criticism, due to a poor "public image," has tended to produce certain withdrawn behavior. But it is becoming apparent that you cannot charge fees sufficient to enable you to meet all the service needs of your patients. Accordingly, the public is becoming aware that you have been asked to be proficient in more different things than any other single person or institution related to the care of disabled individuals. With this is coming the recognition of the necessity for help. As a consequence, most nursing home administrators have been quite willing and have come to know the therapeutic wisdom of having their patients involved with the outside and with outside people. In spite of all of these good intentions, however, and in spite of the use of churches, lodges, and the like, many patients do not respond. They lack motivation. They will not participate in the programs within the homes. They will not get out of their beds. They will not talk, read, or watch television. They will not work. What do you do about all this? First of all, it is absolutely necessary to create an atmosphere of high morale. This is accomplished by active, optimistic programs, by patients being able to leave, go home, or go to other settings. And with this aura, even your bedridden, isolated patients will have the potential of responding to what I am next going to suggest.

The process that I want to briefly describe is called "remotivation technique." You may or may not be familiar with it. It is a technique that has been largely employed in hospital settings with elderly people. While it has been used with psychiatric patients primarily, I want to emphasize that the lack of motivation, regardless of the disease affecting the individual, is a psychological problem and must be approached as such. Remotivation is a technique that can be applied to bed patients, to patients ambulated, or to patients that are mixed in terms of their degree of difficulties or their sex. The only thing patients must have in common is lack of motivation. It is a technique for getting patients to focus their attention on simple objective features of everyday life—things unrelated to their emotional difficulties. The aim is to "remotivate" patients to take a renewed interest in their surroundings.

It is a program that can be readily learned by aides and the inexpensively employed. It is not only a process designed to remotivate patients, it secondarily motivates aide personnel to take greater interest in patients. It was first introduced in 1956 in the Philadelphia State Hospital by the late Dorothy Hoskins Smith. It has spread throughout the country since that time and has been the object of much study. This technique is applied to a group and makes use of one attendant or nurse for one or two hours a week. Therefore, it takes minimal personnel for a large number of people.

A group may, of course, be quite small or it may have as many as ten people. The technique of remotivation consists of a series of meetings held once or twice a week under the leadership of some home person. Usually the series consists of twelve sessions. Patients are encouraged to take part, but are not forced. Each meeting lasts from thirty minutes to an hour. Each time the leader guides the discussion through five specific steps. First he creates a *Climate of Acceptance.* He moves around the group of patients, who may be in a circle, speaking to each one individually and expressing appreciation to each for attending. He encourages each patient to reply by commenting on the weather, some familiar or pleasant incident or the patient's dress. Next, objective poetry is used to create a *Bridge to the World.* As he reads, the leader circles the seated group and then urges each patient in turn, if possible, to read a brief passage from the poem. He asks questions to stimulate discussion of the idea expressed in the poem. In Step 3, *Sharing the World We Live In,* objective questions by the leader develop the subject further. Concrete objects and often such things as drawings, maps, and live animals are used to promote interest and to make the subject more real. Step 3 merges into Step 4, *The Work of the World,* in which the patient is encouraged to talk about work in relation to himself, to tell how a particular job is done or to talk about the kind of work he likes. In the fifth and last step, the leader creates a *Climate of Appreciation;* he thanks each patient for participating and discusses plans for the next meeting to give the patients a sense of continuity and expression. This simple procedure helps establish the warm and understanding relationship and the combination of appreciation, trust, and respect for another human being which is the foundation of mental health.

A few additional comments may clarify this program a bit further. First of all, materials used in these programs can be obtained easily from libraries, friends' homes, or made by you. In planning the timing of these meetings, it has been suggested that the first step, the Climate of Acceptance, take five minutes; the second, third, and fourth steps each take fifteen minutes, and the final step, the Climate of Appreciation, take five. One usually draws up a plan prior to the meeting. An example might be such as this:

Step 1, the Climate of Acceptance: Speak to each person individually and express appreciation for his coming.

Step 2, Bridge to the World: "What kinds of animals are found in Africa?" (Several answers given until someone says tiger.) "What does a tiger look like?" (Allow for some descriptions and then show pictures of tigers.) And then the poem, *The Tiger* (William Blake), is read by the group.

Step 3, Sharing the World We Live In: "Why are men afraid of tigers?" "What other animals are fearful?" "What else is Africa famous for?" (List several other related questions.)

Step 4, The Work of the World: "What products come from Africa?" (A number of answers will lead to a discussion of work and jobs in Africa. Show pictures from *National Geographic* of African diamond mines, Egyptian cotton and oil, etc.)

Step 5, Climate of Appreciation: Thank patients for coming and express pleasure at the quality of this meeting and plan for the next.

When one becomes interested in doing this it is necessary that he study the available literature. Opportunities are open for taking short courses, if desired, in conducting this type of program. It is important for the remotivator to begin with a group he feels will make some type of good response so that confidence can be gained by the experience and discouragement avoided. Remember, you may become quite frustrated if you pick out the most hopeless situations at first. The more severely regressed patients should be left until later on, after the program is further developed. Also, if the remotivator is unable to get responses from some of the patients, it is possible to ask other patients to attempt to get responses and participation.

If you are motivated to explore this procedure further, I suggest you write to the American Psychiatric Association, Mental Hospital Service, The SK & F Foundation, Remotivation Project, Box 7929, Philadelphia 1, Pennsylvania. It has to be remembered that this technique is capable of bringing an individual out of his isolated world and the program cannot stop here. Other programs must take up from this point.

Let me branch off again and make a few other observations. It is helpful to recognize that the emotional problems of your elderly patients are not any different from those of younger people. Remember that aging is not a disease. It does not have to mean emotional and mental deterioration. It doesn't have to mean "second childhood." We must approach disease in the older person in the same fashion as we approach it in the younger—always aware that catastrophe may occur, cognizant of limitations, but consistently optimistic.

You might ask, "Is not senility a disease of age?" I say it is a disease that occurs in the older individual, but it has not been proven to be a disease of the aging process itself. Let me assure you that psychiatric disorders associated with the elderly show as much reversibility as in the younger, even with massive brain damages. Even though we have considered for many years symptoms of senile arteriosclerotic brain disease, such as short memory, disorientation, emotional lability, thinking difficulties, and poor judgment to be the direct result of brain damage, postmortem studies have tended to prove that symptoms expressed during the lifetime correlate very little with the amount of brain damage actually found. And thus, the spry, elderly, active person, age ninety, being involved until the very moment of the final coma, may, at autopsy, be found to be riddled with cancer or severe brain damage, while the older debilitated, sick, forgetful, uninvolved person may be found to have a surprisingly well-intact brain. Anxiety, irritability, timidity, and other personality changes frequently seen in senility are not attributable solely to changes in the brain, but are probably due to the individual's being shoved into a position that frustrates his wishes and deprives him of his usefulness and of his status as an autonomous person. A failure to find the satisfactions necessary to replace those the elderly person had when he felt needed, important, and productive, tends to lead to regressive changes.

Many of us, in order to prolong life, operate with the philosophy that if we have an opportunity to stand still, why not sit down, and if we can sit down, why not lie down, and if we can lie down, why not sleep for a while? I have been suggesting that the opposite attitude must be assumed and that rehabilitative thoughts must be applied to every patient in your homes. If they are alive and lying down, why can't they sit up, and if they are sitting up, why can't they stand up, and if they can stand up, why can't they walk, and if they can walk, why can't they go some place, and if they go some place, why can't they do something? Yes, I know about the patient who has been recently admitted to your home suffering from the terminal stage of cancer, and I know the doctor has told you the patient will die soon. I also know that this prediction is often wrong and that if you accept it without question, your rehabilitative efforts will be proportional and minimal.

Only the first step has been taken when nursing homes have excellent basic programs in operation. A vital second step remains. I refer here to consistent rehabilitative effort. Traditionally, rehabilitation has been conceptualized almost entirely in terms of the needs of younger people. Despite the many excellent programs and all the volunteer help which has been enlisted, the efforts are yet insufficient. Most of you rely upon the family doctor to be equipped to counsel you and treat your patients for all ailments. Most of you must come to the realization that this is not possible for any one person to do. Energetic programs must involve constant reevaluations of your patients' difficulties. This involves consultations with specialists who have hospital facilities. In our community, if I were to believe that the incidence of emotional difficulties in a local nursing home is directly proportional to the number of consultations we are asked to make, I would conclude that there are few or no problems. Our facilities are seldom used by nursing homes and, therefore, consultation almost never exists. One consultation I cited earlier in my presentation may be an example of what you can do for some of your patients. You may attend meetings and have techniques explained, but I have long since learned that in the teaching of physicians and medical students, the instruction must be built around specific problems in specific patients, at the time they are occurring. Only in this way can you really learn the meaning behind these words.

SUMMARY

With these thoughts in mind, I would offer the following summary of observations on coping with the emotional problems of elderly patients:

1. Resentment of outside help and "healthy interference" means stagnation and restricted programs.

2. Specialists should be asked to make periodic reevaluations of your patients' illnesses and problems. It is lethal to assume that

any chronic problem need have only one evaluation, one prognostic statement, and one course of treatment.

3. Severe and acute emotional problems can best be handled by judicious use of proper medications.

4. Emotional problems of all people, as well as the aged, are best handled by their prevention. It is false to presume that the aged have any problems quite different from those of any other age group.

5. What I have called the acquisition of technical skills, is well on its way to full establishment. But a second step, involving rehabilitative goals for the elderly in nursing homes, is yet to be attained.

6. The one mechanism that is going to do the most to prevent emotional problems from developing is *adequate preparation of the patients for entrance* into your home and your program.

7. All programs in the treatment of illness and related problems are premised on the idea that healthy parts remain, and that it is utilization of these parts which allows us to overcome the problems.

8. It is necessary to establish programs that are calculated to meet all of the humanistic needs that have existed through the years, prior to becoming aged and debilitated.

9. Don't forget that patients may respond to those whom they perceive as being more like them. Therefore, do make use of the willing efforts of other patients.

10. For the unmotivated patients, try the remotivation technique. Send for the literature, read it, and only then make the decision as to whether you can use it and whether it will work.

And finally, none of us, alone, can cope with the problems of human beings. It takes all our efforts together—those of the patient and his relatives and friends, volunteers, the family physician, clergymen, community organizations, hospitals, aides, nurses, and, especially, the full, perceptive efforts of the only person who can pull this therapeutic team together, the nursing home administrator.

Chapter 3

Trends in Care

JEROME KAPLAN

> Now in building of chaises, I tell you what,
> There is always somewhere a weakest spot . . .
> And that's the reason, beyond a doubt,
> That a chaise breaks down, but doesn't wear out.
>
> — OLIVER WENDELL HOLMES

As of today, aging remains an enigma. We can talk ourselves slowly around the periphery of the subject, replying to pointed queries here and there, but the answer to the crucial question, "What is it?" eludes us.

Perhaps curious man has always wondered why some people in their eighties are physically and intellectually vigorous whereas others decline considerably by the age of sixty years. Although it is difficult to say when the search for an answer to this riddle began, it is even less clear when or how it will end.

Two sciences that deal particularly with problems of aging have evolved: (1) geriatrics, which focuses on the diseases of old age, and (2) gerontology, which is chiefly concerned with the process of aging. Geriatrics takes a clinical approach and makes therapeutic use of the knowledge at hand; gerontology seeks the benefits of new concepts in preventive medicine.

Through research, we are learning how changes in social and health status affect old people. New theories are evolving and earlier ones are being substantiated or modified. These theories, in turn, are the basis for the present and future evolvement of appropriate social institutions. Social institutions are creations of the community and of its citizen actions and interactions. Aging, as an individual and social phenomenon, is a major force for change in the basic organization of social life. Its effects on the basic social institutions through which human effort is channeled and by which biological, psychological, and social need is achieved, is now being only imperfectly understood.

The organization and content of health and social services are significant areas of community life which are responding to this fact of aging. The majority of the responses and resultant changes, however, have been spontaneous and unplanned. Only a few such services have, in reality, been the result of planned change.

The community must assume greater responsibilities toward old people, not only for their well-being but for its own. The later years of life should be a fruitful period of growth and improvement in mind and character, a time of continued contributions by the old people to better themselves and their communities. A well-planned program within the community should try to anticipate those problematic situations which may confront the elderly and their families. These include potential deterioration of personality and character, loss of self-esteem, and withdrawal from the satisfactions of everyday living. One means to avert these effects is positive control of the environment in which older people live.

LEISURE AND RETIREMENT

Age forces change upon old people, and successful adjustment to aging demands changes in every sphere of activity. Although some relaxation of activity may be necessary, mental and physical health can be maintained only through self-discipline. However, the older person must find or be provided with circumstances favorable to that maintenance. He may find he has time on his hands after he has passed the age when he is expected to give up his major social and personal responsibilities (and self-discipline is dependent on having responsibilities to meet).

Anyone who makes a sudden break from one way of life to another without adequate preparation often finds great difficulties of adjustment, and old people are subject to great distress because of the worries peculiar to old age. Ill health, fear of death, loss of relatives and friends, poor or inadequate housing, fear of losing work, financial insecurity or a reduced income, and their children's and the public's indifference are part of their lengthy list of woes. The aging person may make a favorable adjustment to his altered situation when, given good health, he is still able to be productive at work or at home, but, in addition to work, the older person must be capable of finding release from his burdens through leisure.

Retirement suddenly presents a great amount of leisure. That leisure which was once merely a period of refreshment must now become an end in itself. The recognition, status, prestige, self-expression, and friendship once afforded by work must now be derived from leisure.

The average American, however, lives in a culture that consciously manifests a distrust and suspicion of leisure; he is imbued with a puritanical faith that life without work is meaningless. But the traditional values of the past can only cause dislocation if they are not revised to be in keeping with present-day facts. Today, an ever-increasing consumer expenditure is for leisure activity. The seventy-hour work week has been reduced to a forty-hour, and a thirty-hour work week has been envisaged in some industries. For a person without household tasks—for example, patients in nursing homes and residents of homes for the aged—the whole day is leisure time.

Adjustment to retirement can be aided in part by becoming psychologically prepared for it. A further part, of course, involves the attitude and conception of what constitutes a worthwhile role. How leisure activity or recreation is defined by the older person is important. Some older people insist they are so active as volunteers or as members of an organization that they have no time for leisure. This was borne out by a sixty-eight-year-old man, retired for three years, who insisted he spent so much time working around his house, watching television, and taking an active part in a retirement club that he had no leisure time. For others, leisure-time pursuits represent the uselessness to which society has relegated them. For example, retirement from work is difficult to accept as a normal phase of life by some farmers. This is readily understandable, since retirement then conflicts with their social values of usefulness and productivity.

The older person clings to a tradition of culture in which work is all-important and in which success and achievement are correlated with work. A part of this tradition connects growth with the young. Hence, programs for people must give them a chance to realize growth through leisure and through recreational activities. New meanings for leisure must be discovered. This statement has significant connotations for nursing homes and homes for the aged for it suggests that recreation and therapy programs must be considered as significant as dietary and nursing functions and must be related not only to the overall subculture of the groups served but also to the very specific requirements of each person as an individual. Ways must be found by which persons can contribute their free time to their community and this contribution be held in respect and dignity even though it is not one of work.

Although organization is the rule in almost every phase of modern life, retirement is entered upon without adequate planning or thought. The relinquishment of work and the beginning of retirement bring about significant changes in daily routine and a possible disruption of social relationships. An appropriate understanding of leisure may preserve dignity and respect for the older person even when his social status has changed.

THE YOUNG AND THE OLD

A review of history shows that old people are most secure when society has developed a mutually supportive and intermingled relationship between the old and the young. Youth and age do much to complement and inspire each other. When specific activities for only the old are outlined, the proper relationship of these activities to youth should not be forgotten. For example, any program developed in a home for the aged should recognize occasionally the zest and enthusiasm which can be brought only by children and adolescents.

Often we forget the kindness, wisdom, and stories which the elders can bring to the young. There is no absolute substitute for the common interests which bind youth and age together. Although this is true, there are synthetics which, at times, serve to supplement and, if necessary, replace the "genuine article." Foster homes, the Golden Age recreation movement, aid to geriatric patients, and retirement counseling are only a small portion of the programs now under way.

Far oftener than is necessary or desirable, older persons are denied opportunities to share and contribute as much as they could or should. Ours is a culture which tends to exclude older people and emphasize opportunities for the young.

COMMUNITY ATTITUDES

Just as the individual must face the changes introduced by older years, so must the community prepare for its older citizens. Each community must learn to produce an environment conducive to desirable changes. The America of today carries with it an attitude of ambivalence toward the older people and the aged. On one hand, they are regarded as figures of authority; on the other, as dependent and childlike.

An individual is seldom responsible for defining his place in the sun. Part of the social battle and part of the person's internal conflict arise from the gap between what an older person is allowed to do, what he is able to do, and what he thinks he can do. This kind of uncertainty is found more frequently in societies in transition that have not been able to prescribe different types of roles for persons in specific age categories. Feelings of security, prestige, and opportunities for participation and interaction are dependent upon what a community considers normal at a particular time.

In a rapidly changing society, the opportunity for active participation by the old is disrupted. Rapid social change tends to inactivate the older person, while stable conditions may set the pattern of participation by him. Seniority rights aptly illustrate the latter; being overlooked by an organization which one has served faithfully in the past or suddenly being given an honorary membership to replace an active one, are examples of the former. More often than necessary, the effects are devastating, for what is a well-intentioned act serves to cut older people off from the rest of the group. Henceforth, they are "different."

More factors than one undoubtedly influence change within an individual. Yet, more and more, a person is considered old by his community when he loses his social competence, whether it be from individual failure or through community apathy.

On the other hand, the ways numerous subcultural groups deal with the aged or work with older persons have not been fully explored. Successful aging rests upon the capacity of the older person to take advantage of opportunities made available to him by the society of which he is a part. In our society, it is grossly difficult to equate with old age the values of prestige, respect, or the material securities. In the eyes of the community, few roles are reserved for the old to be performed with dignity or with prestige. Even the grandparent baby-sitter is not rated as highly as the young baby-sitter. More and more, older people in our society experience contractions in social relationships as their work group and family group become either substantially altered or nonexistent.

Playing a role in the productive economy or within the household, when coupled with good health, is predictive of a favorable adjustment to aging. On the other hand, the family structure is less and less a unit except for parents and their young children. The present emphasis is upon the conjugal, or one- or two-generation family, which, by definition, precludes aged parents. The scattered family has become an accepted part of the "New America." Occupation or selection of another part of the country for various reasons lure many away forever from the parental home. The social roles of the adult in the family unit are altered and, in some instances, are changed from provider and housekeeper to dependent.

Isolation and loneliness are potential creators of problems. Loneliness comes when family group relationships are greatly modified without compensatory relationships to take their place. Yet, as adults grow older, social relationships other than those associated with daily work activities are progressively restricted to relatives. We expect the young to break away from the old and the old not to live with the young, although an unmarried daughter may feel a psychologic push or be actually pressured by the married siblings to care for the old parent. More often than not, the traditional three-generation family in the United States causes conflict rather than harmony. A new type of family relationship of independence of both the older and younger generations has sprung up.

Although the social roles of persons in family units change with age, an increase in status, respect, or security is not always insured. It is good to cheer the older person and the aged by pleasant labels, by exaggeration of work capacity, by assurance of happy retirement years, and by minimizing biologic quiescence. However, both personal and community planning must face realism as to health, income, housing, social relations, status, and adjustment. Unrealistic optimism breeds disillusion and neglect.

Aging, to be personally acceptable, must allow older people to find places in society whereby they believe they are participating strategically. How a nursing home is used by an individual and how he is helped to use a nursing home when indicated is crucial to the acceptability of aging.

CHALLENGE TO PLANNING

Total community planning needs to give more consideration to its entire organizational structure. The variance between that which is socially expected and that which is socially available is a tremendous challenge. Although our efforts toward helping older people adjust to personal problems should not be abated, an immense effort should be exerted to eliminate the lack of opportunities within society which precipitate many individual difficulties.

The loss of associations which have disintegrated must be replaced with other equally satisfactory group associations. The views and actions of the older person are greatly dependent on how useful he feels in relation to his surroundings. Is this not a challenge to the nursing home for at least some patients? It is difficult to realize that in old age there is at last time for intellectual, cultural, and spiritual activities. Only in very recent years has society through its collective organizations begun to guide older people and the aged to a full life in the later years.

It is important to older people to remain active participants in group affairs in either operational or supervisory roles. The other basic concerns of older people, such as a long life, protection from the hazards of living, safeguarding or strengthening the prerogative of seniority, and a comfortable and honorable withdrawal from life when physical necessity requires it, are constant permeating influences as the community makes opportunities available to elderly people.

Community planning geared to older persons' needs is basic for the urban community, the small town, and the rural environment. Regardless of geography, a concerted community effort is necessary. The older person may be just as isolated and discontented in a small community as in a city, in a small nursing home as in a large home for the aged. We have been holding onto a sentimental belief that the small community is an ideal place to live in the later years of life. While long-established small communities in the United States have more older people proportionately than the larger cities, it is probably due in large measure to the migration of the young and to the reluctance of homeowners to move. This does not underestimate the importance of social ties but suggests other factors which cut down movement by many older people.

When the husband or wife dies or when they are estranged, when the children move, when the number of old friends declines rapidly, and when there is no longer a job, the older person exists on the periphery of life rather than in the center of social relationships. He cannot turn to his mate, his children, or old friends. The number of friends an older person thinks he has may even be at variance with the opinion of those he considers his friends. This is a major factor limiting opportunities for informal participation. Consequently, any efforts directed toward individual adjustment must also be concerned with the opportunities available within our communities. We are faced with a twofold challenge of great magnitude: preparing the individual to adjust and accept his changing role within society and providing the climate and sources that allow new senior roles.

Community planning on all levels must learn how to develop the basic resources. In addition to reaching old people who dwell in independent households, it must recognize the relationships introduced by aged people who live in concentrated areas. We must learn how to create stimulating and effective environments for those residing within and without the institution. Through intelligent action programs we must learn to discern between problems caused essentially by the personality of an individual and those caused by the personality of the community, such as the physical environment of a building, the philosophy of an administrator, or the actions of a staff.

Certain prerequisites for an adequate program for the rural older people and the aged are largely beyond the scope of local community action *only*. In this category fall the need for retirement and health benefit systems; additional attention to the employment needs of older people in state employment services; more adequate old age assistance payments when needed; additional adequate medical facilities, including nursing homes; basic and practical research in all phases of aging; demonstration and pilot projects; and fellowships and stipends for continuous learning and training.

PROFILE OF PATIENTS

It is necessary to understand the characteristics of the persons who seek out and reside in nursing homes and homes for the aged. These characteristics provide the basis for the types of structures and the total diet-nursing-therapeutic complex of such homes. Some of these are:

1. Most of the residents lived formerly in the same geographic area where the nursing home or home for the aged is located.
2. Most of them have relatives in the same area even though there are some without relatives.
3. Most of them are elderly, seventy-five years of age and over.
4. Women residents outnumber men by about three to one.
5. Most admissions are arranged by relatives.
6. Most of the residents are functionally disabled with a growing number that are confused in one or more areas.

7. Most of them enter nursing homes and homes for the aged to remain indefinitely.

No doubt many persons are admitted because of social deprivations, lack of family support, and forceful pushing by old age aid investigators. This raises questions about the ability of the helping professions as well as of the larger community to perceive the need for community alternatives to institutional placements when family or traditional living arrangements no longer provide for the safety and security of older individuals. The fact that few persons after admission to such facilities are expected to return to the community, raises questions as to the goals and the effectiveness of the services provided. The fact that in late winter 1964, approximately 80 per cent (close to 1,100) of all nursing homes in Ohio were cited as having electrical wiring deficiencies, raises the further question of whether the physical plants are safe.

ADMINISTRATORS' SELF-EVALUATION

For those about to begin administration or those who have recently entered the field, it is necessary to face a self-evaluation. All gerontological professionals should do this, anyway, periodically. Some of the more pertinent questions and possible answers follow:

Q. Why do some people become discouraged in administering to chronically ill persons, especially the elderly?

A. I have observed, as have others, that not all administrators are capable of dealing with large numbers of chronically ill persons with sustained enthusiasm. A number of my colleagues have devoted some attention to this problem, and my thoughts are clearly influenced by their investigations. The administrator, like all other people, if he is to live and work effectively, must maintain his self-esteem. The administrator's evaluation of himself as an individual capable of reducing or eliminating stress and restoring and/or maintaining faith is apt to suffer when he cannot see clearly the patients' improvement as the result of his efforts. The administrator's self-esteem is also very much influenced by how much he is liked and appreciated by his patients. The chronically ill patient who is frustrated by his slow progress is not likely to express gratitude to the administrator for his help. In fact, the patient frequently might indicate that he is dissatisfied. Another complication is that the administrator may not be fully aware of the changes going on within the psyche of the chronically ill patient. The administrator may recognize many psychosocial complications, but since he may not have a complete grasp of each of these complications, it is exceedingly difficult to locate methods of coping with them. This, in turn, adds to feelings of not doing "all I can."

You might ask why this difficulty may be exaggerated in the elderly person who is chronically ill. Undoubtedly, the special problems of elderly persons have many facets, but the psychosocial complications for the elderly patient are often extremely complex. In addition, one cannot ignore the fact that the older patient is considered to be a threat by some members of the various professional service disciplines. Usually it is an unconscious threat; a sick, very old person reminds us that eventually all of us will decline and die.

Q. What can be done to fortify the administrator against discouragement?

A. The administrator can be made to function more effectively if he understands himself and his patient. For example, it is wise for an administrator to understand the so-called "sick role" in our society. In our society the "sick role" is acceptable to the individual and to the group, if it is a temporary condition. The chronic occupancy of the "sick role" produces many distortions and maladjustments. Some people actually use it as a refuge. A hypochondriac is such a person. Other people prefer to remain in the "sick role" when it offers some situational advantage. Administrators should be aware of the cases of "hospitalitis" and those who are reluctant to give up disability pensions. Society, in turn, is apt to reject the chronically impaired individual who does not "overcome" his handicap and in some manner make a contribution to society. Although perhaps not always consistent with Judeo-Christian ideals, an insistence that a sick person make a contribution to society is often necessary for his own good. The individual who is hospitalized or immobilized for any length of time discovers that he is "out of it." His family and friends adjust their lives so that they can carry on without the patient's participation. The vacancy he has created in social affairs by his illness is filled by a new participant. If this pattern of living is maintained for any length of time, the living habits of the family become firmly established and are resistant to change. In fact, it is not unusual for the family to discover that it is easier in some respects to deal independently of the chronically ill person, since it eliminates from consideration his possibly divergent viewpoint. It is no wonder that when a person improves to the point that he tries to find his way back into his family and circle of friends, he encounters considerable resistance. Clearly, the chronically ill person has a number of handicaps to overcome. He must struggle against physical impairment and psychosocial difficulties. To reduce at least one of these handicaps, the administrator and the patient must consistently and realistically appraise the social situation.

Q. What support should the administrator ask of the patient's family?

A. The administrator may wish to urge the patient's family and friends not to close their circle against the patient but insist that they preserve a place for him by maximizing communication with the patient and having the patient participate in important decisions, assuming basic mental functions are still preserved.

Q. What other reactions should the administrator expect from chronically ill persons?

A. The chronically ill patient resents his physical illness and the psychosocial experiences forced upon him. Chronically ill persons react in a number of ways to lack of progress. Some withdraw and accept the "sick role." Others become depressed, but not infrequently they became irritable and angry. Feelings of anger are apt to be aimed at those responsible for their care. They will express the feeling that the administrator and other members of the treatment team are incompetent and disinterested. It is essential that the nursing home staff understand that this reaction to frustration is an expected one and that they should accept it without retaliating or arguing.

When intense hostility is held in check, it gradually builds up and becomes a highly destructive force within the patient. When such dammed-up feelings are given expression, the disruptive element is reduced, and the energies of the patient can be directed into constructive efforts.

Q. Is there any way an administrator can tell when he and his staff are successfully coping with the emotional complications of chronic illness?

A. The administrator has several methods of evaluating the success of his efforts. Of prime importance is the response of the patient. If the patient does not retreat from his personal and social responsibility and if he maintains his self-respect by seeking and establishing new patterns of adjustment, the administrator knows he has succeeded. I want to reemphasize that it is important for *both* patient and administrator to maintain their self-esteem. The patient, in order to overcome much of his physical disability, must feel respected by others and believe that he is contributing to their lives and well-being. The administrator can measure his success as the leader of a team through the increased professional satisfaction he obtains from dealing effectively with the chronically ill.

These, then, are philosophical concepts and general principles of the current trends in the care of the aged. The total community approach and its resources and how they are used relate to this type of care given within the nursing home–home for the aged constellation. The milieu for the latter includes a comprehensive therapeutic concept relating to the total needs of each of its patients through appropriate programs as indicated earlier.

Within a decade the nursing or retirement home which does not heed certain signs of changing care trends is doomed. There must be greater acceptance and use of professionally organized homemaker and home care services; out-patient and day care services; acceptance of the concept of rehabilitation for the elderly; enlarged meals-on-wheels services; apartment type housing, including public housing with medical clinics; retirement housing with infirmary units, as typically provided by churches and fraternal organizations; increased emphasis upon a professional degree requirement for administrators; cooperative relationship and/or affiliation with a general hospital, among others. The gradual growth of nursing home type "wings" attached to general hosiptals will become a major challenge to the "independent" nursing home. In other words, the nursing or retirement home must become an integral part of this total scheme to serve the chronically ill and the elderly. Otherwise, it cannot morally be considered as serving humanity in an appropriate manner, nor can it, in reality, so serve.

The challenge is now here. As in the building of a chaise—as stated by Oliver Wendell Holmes—there is always a weakest spot, as there is in the care of the aged. Perhaps these comments will help to develop and to maintain quality of patient care so that the chaise—or the right kind of service at the proper point of time—will not "break down."

Part Two

POLICIES AND PROCEDURES IN ADMINISTRATION

Chapter 4

Building and Executing a Patient Care Plan

ALTON E. BARLOW

The dramatic and acute short-term illnesses have long claimed the major attention of professional groups and the general public. Chronic illness, which is the reason the majority of patients are in congregate living settings, has been neglected in consequence. Attention to acute phases of chronic illness has tended to be transient and minimal and professional services to the long-term patient have often been meager. However, during the past decade we have seen this situation changing. What are some of the reasons for such change?

1. Changes in our living pattern. We have developed a culture which accents youth, while at the same time we are adding millions of older persons to our population. In 1900 the life expectancy was 47 years; it rose to 68 in 1950, and is now 70.3 years. Many of the aged are ill and not infrequently require almost constant and highly specialized care. Not all, of course, are aged. In fact 16 per cent of the chronically ill are under 25. There are 1,600,000 complete invalids in this country.

2. Many present-day families are not financially able to provide care for the chronically sick and aged member. Moreover, the small houses and apartments in vogue today more often than not do not include the "extra room" for grandmother. Even if such a room were available, with both husband and wife working, who would care for the aged person?

3. Many of our general hospitals, and especially our mental hospitals, are overcrowded. A large proportion of those who are old and ill do not need the battery of services provided in a general hospital and those who most need it probably cannot afford it.

4. The influence of a mass geriatric population on a national

culture is without precedent. The United States will be the first country to confront and accommodate the social and economic changes set in motion by an aged population which has passed the 18,000,000 mark and will nearly double by the turn of the century.

5. The problems of the aged have become a familiar target of the politician. Congress is likely to respond favorably to the special political urgency of enacting programs for older persons, even though the planners may not agree as to what kinds of programs would be most acceptable.

6. More and more, groups which have become interested in the care of the chronically ill and aged are making increased demands for information.

Because of these pressures and the fact that care of the chronically ill is difficult at best, there will always be the need for nursing homes. How these nursing homes are operated and by whom depends a great deal on the attitudes of the present-day administrators. The mere fact that administrators are increasingly participating in conferences and short courses proves their desire to add to their competence in dealing with the many facets of nursing home administration. This participation reflects also their determination to be part of the new and broader concept in nursing home care.

It is incumbent upon all institutions to see that their policies and practices are carefully framed and meticulously carried out in the interest of the patient. Most important among these are admission and discharge policies.

No institution should admit a patient whose essential care requirements it is not prepared to meet. Therefore, prior to admission, you should carefully screen the patient in terms of kind and nature of care necessary, type of emotional problems present, and special physical conditions (such as incontinence or mental deterioration). You should screen also for ability to pay the price you must charge in your facility. It is easier to move a patient from a four-bed accommodation to a private room than to reverse the procedure.

At this time, also, settle the financial transaction and obtain a signed admission agreement. It is wise to provide the interested relative with a copy of this agreement. Fix the fee in advance and discuss variations from the basic rate which may be needed, if the basic condition becomes worse and additional care is required. Agree as to who pays for the extras and how. List the types of extras and the approximate cost, so the relative will have some idea of the additional monthly expenses. Agree as to pharmacy charges. Does the relative have a pharmacy of preference? Should billing be directly from the pharmacy or through the nursing home? If the patient must be taken to another place for specialized services who does the transporting and is there a charge? Define your visiting hours, if you observe them, and your policy in regard to patient visiting outside the institution. By all means, discuss completely your policy in regard to refund arrangements in the event of death or transfer to another facility, and the amount of prior notice for a change in rate or for discharge of the patient.

At this time you should obtain the name of the physician who will care for the patient and include in your admission agreement permission for your house physician to care for the patient in the event you cannot reach his own doctor. You should inquire about recent hospitalization of the patient and obtain written permission for release of information so you may obtain a transcript from the hospital. Again, it is most important that you have your admission agreement signed by the responsible party and that you make a copy of such agreement available to this person.

WELCOMING THE PATIENT

The admission of the patient is particularly important because it is at the admission desk that a new resident, often acutely sensitive to every cue about the place, gains an initial impression of what the facility will be like. This one brief experience may set the tone for acceptance or rejection of what is to come.

The majority of patients admitted to nursing homes go directly to their beds and frankly are emotionally and/or physically exhausted by the move from one living situation to another. Their primary concern is how and whom to call to attend to their basic needs. It is important for the admitting nurse to show the new patient the call system and, if the patient is allowed to ambulate, the location of the bathroom. It is also important that such personal effects as toilet articles be within easy reach. For such a patient the second or even third day is time enough to learn about food preferences and during the ensuing week time can be taken to discover the range of activities within the patient's capabilities.

The ambulant or wheelchair (self-propelled) patient may be acclimated to the new situation in a different manner. The admitting nurse, or in a larger institution possibly the activities director, may introduce the new resident to his fellow patients, the attendants, and nursing staff. The patient should be made to feel he has been expected and wanted. The welcome can be rounded out by showing the patient about the building and grounds and encouraging participation in a game or discussion with older residents. These techniques of welcome, as well as others that will occur to you, will turn out to be of considerable importance in promoting the rapid participation of the new arrival in the patient community.

Each new patient should receive an admission bath at which time the nurse should note any bruises or unusual body conditions which may require special care. This is protection for you against blame for a preexisting condition. The admitting nurse or an aide should make a list of the personal possessions accompanying the patient and make certain each item is properly marked or identified.

TRANSFER OR DISCHARGE OF THE PATIENT

Just as a nursing home should not admit a patient unless it is prepared to meet essential care requirements, it should not continue to care for the patient whose condition has improved sufficiently for return to community living, or the patient whose condition has worsened and who now requires a higher degree of service than the institution is prepared to render.

Let us first consider the patient who has improved. Your first step should be discussion with the physician of the improvement in the patient's condition and the poor effect that remaining in an institutional setting of "sick" people can have on the accomplished gains. After obtaining the physician's consent, you should discuss the transfer with the responsible relative. Make sure you have some boarding home in mind, should the family prefer not to return the patient to his own home. Having obtained the cooperation of the family, you must now find out what the patient wants to do. Explain why the move is in the best interest of all concerned and give reassurance that you are not trying to "get rid" of the patient. In some cases it may be important to give reassurance of prompt readmission to your home, should the need arise. When the final decision has been reached, provide the family with information, in writing, on the diet and medication essentials. Supply them with a patient care plan—that is, what has been done for the patient at what times. Mention the limitations with regard to self-help, activities, rest periods, etc. You must show the family what it takes to keep the patient from losing the gains or improvements you have helped him to accomplish. When the time of actual discharge arrives try to make it an occasion. Have the patient dress in his finest. Be sure that all personal possessions are ready and itemized, and that ample time is provided for farewells to other patients. Again, give reassurance of your willingness to readmit the patient to the home, should the need arise.

If the patient is going to a facility offering lesser care, such as a boarding home or rest home, it is even more important that you follow all the steps outlined. Of course, patients are often moved to another nursing home because the family or patient is dissatisfied with the service rendered by your facility. This does not lessen your responsibility to supply the information necessary for the patient's continued care.

Transfer to a hospital can be a greater emotional shock for the patient. If the patient's mental and physical condition permits, the reasons for the transfer should be carefully explained with emphasis on the short-term treatment phase of the planned hospitalization and the hoped-for speedy return to your facility. You should send, with the patient, a card with the name and address of the responsible relative, the physician who has cared for the patient at your home, the patient's name, date of birth, birthplace, and, if a public assistance case, the name and address of the responsible agency and the assistance number. Since most transfers to a hospital are made on a physician's orders, it is assumed that a brief medical history will be supplied by the referring physician.

FORMAL ACCOUNTING

Whether a patient has been transferred to a general hospital, a lesser care facility, or has died, the final step as an ending to your transaction with this patient should be handled in a businesslike fashion. Give the responsible person a formal accounting of the financial status of the patient account, showing all charges and credits. Collect all the monies due your institution or make a refund and give documentary receipts of the transaction. In some cases when the patient has been in a facility for some time the family may wish to have any refund allocated to a patient fund or divided among the staff members. If such is the case, be sure you have such intention clearly stated in writing as well as a record of how you allocated the funds. Should the patient's clothing be left for you to dispose of, a similar written notification should be obtained.

MEDICAL AND NURSING CARE

Institutions must beware of the thinking behind assertions that a particular program is "good for the patients." Because of the difference in human beings, such generalizations are not necessarily true. A particular program may answer the needs of some patients and be quite unsuited to others. A service required by one patient may be contraindicated for another with the same diagnosis. Thus, we need a patient care plan. The key to a patient care plan is individualized services with flexibility which stems from a realization that the needs of individuals do differ and change with time and circumstances. A patient care plan cannot be a static thing. A care plan made at the time of admission frequently prevents further deterioration and can create a rehabilitation climate for the staff which is essential to good care.

The first step in the program must be working with the physician. You should be guided by the diagnosis and the physician's orders. Within this limitation you may plan for the first efforts toward self-care. We all know it is often easier to do everything for a patient than to take the time to help the patient do it himself. However, are we being fair to the patient? The more you do the more you are encouraging your patients to become like infants. Even if only partial self-care is possible, using that part may be the means of preserving the patient's independence and dignity as a human being. Set a goal; when that has been reached set another.

As part of your care plan write out what each patient is able to do and to what extent. What "tricks" have you been able to teach him to help attain greater ease in performing these activities? What blocks does the patient have in regard to particular activities and what is especially enjoyable? If you are to achieve the maximum potential from your plan you must have the majority of the nursing care staff working with the patient in as near uniform methods as possible. Bladder and bowel retraining is only achieved by concerted effort at the same time daily. So it is with a patient's rehabilitation potential. The patient must want to improve. The staff, other patients, and family members can help by commenting on each gain and minimizing each setback.

Nursing Staff

Who should formulate this patient care plan? Logically, it is the nursing care staff. This brings us to our next problem—what about personnel in nursing homes and what is a nursing care staff?

We believe that improvement of institutional care depends to a great extent on the quality of personnel. It is especially important to have personnel standards that attract able people and assure a measure of job security. Patients are upset by constant staff changes. Naturally, in a nursing home, the nursing care staff, as the group with the greatest degree of direct patient contact, should have the greatest degree of competence.

The nursing care staff consists of the registered nurse, licensed practical nurse, nurse aide, and orderly. Your state licensing authority sets standards as to the amount of licensed nurse personnel and ancillary nursing care staff you are required to maintain. The types of patients you care for and their needs will determine the number of employees, over the licensing requirements, you will have to hire. Failure to provide adequate nursing care personnel will cause your standards of care to suffer. A suggested standard is a minimum of 2½ hours of nursing care per day per patient. Multiplying this by the number of patients cared for and dividing by 8 gives the number of full days of service needed from the nursing home staff per day. If you accept only bed patients a higher ration of nursing care hours would be necessary.

Supervising. Who directs your nursing care staff? As a rule, this varies from the registered professional nurse, or the licensed practical nurse, to the administrator without training. More and more, licensing agencies are adopting the attitude that nursing care should be under the supervision of a registered professional nurse who must be on duty at least forty hours per week. She should be available for consultation at other times.

This means that the registered nurse is the chief of the nursing care team. She supervises the licensed practical nurses and nurse aides. She also makes certain medical judgments and performs specialized treatments. It is the duty of the registered nurse to recognize and interpret symptoms, assist with and institute remedial measures for adverse developments, assist the physician in diagnostic and therapeutic measures and administer medication and treatments as prescribed. She maintains accurate and complete records of nursing observation and care. She must have a genuine interest in geriatric nursing, as well as understanding, patience, and tact in dealing with those under her care. Since she has much contact with patients' relatives, she must likewise be the soul of tact and courtesy. As the leader of the nursing team, she must be able to transmit orders and promote harmony among the nursing care staff.

In many of our smaller institutions, a licensed practical nurse may be in charge of nursing service. She will be expected to assume many of the obligations of the registered nurse. However, she should not assume as much responsibility for making medical judgments or performing certain techniques. Whether a registered nurse or a licensed practical nurse, the leader of the team should not assume responsibility for which she does not have professional competence. She must always rely on the physician for final decision. In large institutions the charge nurse will have little actual patient contact, while in many homes of thirty beds or less she will perform a greater degree of actual bedside care than we have outlined.

The duties of a nurse aide will vary with the size of a facility and the type of patient cared for. She may take temperatures, bathe and feed patients, transport patients from one location to another, comb hair, clean teeth, care for nails, provide bedpans and urinals, make beds and perform some other housekeeping duties. The aide, of course, must report unusual occurrences to the charge nurse and refer all inquiries regarding the patient to the charge nurse or administrator. At no time should she be asked to make independent judgments or to assume responsibility for treatments.

Nursing Procedure Manuals. To assure uniformity of working habits and better patient care every nursing home should have a nursing procedure book. What is contained in this book will depend on the size of the institution and the type of patient cared for. It is suggested that separate procedure manuals be maintained for the professional and nonprofessional staff. In the nonprofessional manual would be outlined such duties as bedmaking, bed bath, A.M. and

P.M. care, care of dentures, giving shampoos (both in and out of bed), positioning of a patient in bed and in a chair, transfer of patient from bed to wheelchair, wheelchair to toilet and back, spoon-feeding, and the like.

The manual for professional or licensed staff would include such items as bladder irrigations and instillations, care of patients in body casts, catheterization, colostomy dressing and irrigation, ear and eye drops, enemas of all types, gastric gavage and lavage, hypodermoclysis, administration of oxygen, abdominal paracentesis, tranfusions, and collection of specimens. Included in both manuals should be a note on professional ethics in the nursing home. It has been stated that uniformity is a curse of a civilized culture but we have found that uniformity in performance leaves little chance for error, and, in our particular field, disturbs the patient less.

Medical Staff

It would appear, in discussing medical and nursing care, that I have put the cart before the horse, since I have left the medical care for last. Your medical profession contacts are by far the most important of any contacts outside your own facility. The physician is, or should be, the focal point around which patient care and planning revolves. He has skills and insight you can't do without. His word is final and he takes the responsibility for being right. It has been suggested recently that nursing homes should have organized medical staffs, much as do the general hospitals. The American Nursing Home Association, American Medical Association, and American Hospital Association, through their tripartite committee, worked on suggested standards for such medical staffs. A guide was published last year and is available through the American Hospital Association. To date few nursing homes have organized a formal staff. However, the reports from those that have, indicate a higher quality of medical supervision and a greater utilization of the nursing homes' potential. We realize it is not possible in many areas to organize a staff.

Each nursing home should have a medical consultant who will assume overall responsibility for the medical care in the nursing home. Select a physician who has an interest in the type patient you care for, who is willing to assist you in the overall medical policy, and who gets along well with other physicians in the area. Such a consultative arrangement does not mean that admission of patients is the exclusive right of this physician. Rather, it gives your facility an expert who is readily available when you need him.

Regardless of what arrangement you make, certain rules must be followed in dealing with the physicians who admit patients to your home. To preserve continuity in patient care, obtain a written medical history from the referring physician or hospital. Always obtain written, signed medical orders. At the time of each patient visit have the physician write a medical progress note and sign it. Obtain your doctor's help in planning patient care, deal ethically with him, and build up the confidence of your patients and staff in his judgments.

Do not allow your staff to overestimate their competence. If they do not understand a physician's order, it is better to ask at the time it is written than to take time from a busy schedule later on. Make sure the physician's orders are always carried out promptly and precisely. In calling a physician be sure an emergency is really an emergency. Have all the information available at the time of visit and thus conserve the physician's time. Your relationship with your doctors may well affect the success of your home.

Hospital Affiliation. I am sure many of you, during the past two years, have heard and read about "hospital affiliation." What is an affiliation? Like an organized medical staff, it is something that has been tried by few nursing homes. The arguments in favor of such arrangements are many. Among these are: prompt hospitalization of patients when needed; better use of facilities through early referrals from the general hospital to the nursing home; better medical supervision; improved public understanding of the long-term care facility; and recognition of the long-term care home as a part of the total health resources of the community. Some feeling exists that the agreement should be a formal, legally binding one, signed by the governing body of the participating facilities.

We say neither arrangement is "right" or "wrong." This is a decision for individual nursing home administrators. However, we suggest it is unrealistic for any general hospital to have such an arrangement with several nursing homes, since it would be spreading its services and supervision rather thinly about the community. We suggest also that most placements in nursing homes are made by families and they still prefer freedom of choice, based usually on financial cost. Admissions from the nursing home to the hospital are, or should be, made by the physicians, so where is the advantage of prompt hospitalization offered through contract? Neither can we envisage any nursing home's being financially able to set aside a number of beds for the exclusive use of one hospital. Such beds are likely to be in no demand at one time and in over demand at another. As I see it, is is more realistic to suggest an informal arrangement between the hospital and the nursing home, where the specialized services of the hospital's staff are available to the nursing home on a fee for service basis, if and when they are not being utilized by the hospital. The nursing home could indicate priority of admission for the hospital's patients, as beds became available. Thus, neither institution would be legally involved and the patient would continue to be served.

Happiness and Well-being of Patients. The happiness and well-being of residents depend far more upon the attitude of management and personnel than on the physical aspects of the building. A safe, sanitary, and comfortable environment is a basic requirement for any facility, but the ability of the staff to provide a cheerful atmosphere and to meet patients' needs is more important. Every home, regardless of size or the degree of infirmity of its residents, needs at least one large living room, accessible to all residents. It should be well lighted and arranged to encourage companionship and activity. In very large facilities it is desirable to have smaller sun parlors or sitting rooms in different areas of the building. If possible, it is helpful and neater to have a separate activity or recreation area. In many of the newer facilities we find that a chapel is enjoyed by the patients.

There is belief in some circles that normal and senile patients should be separated so that both can be happier in the company of others more or less like themselves. It is felt that mentally confused people get along better with each other than when they must compete with persons who can do things better than they. Last year a friend of mine visited a group of nursing homes in England. The homes, all nonprofit, belonged to the same group and varied in size from twenty-four to sixty beds. The president of the organization, a woman with many years' experience in this field, had felt that the confused resident had an adverse effect on the merely physically disabled residents, thus one of the larger homes of forty beds was converted for admission of only the disoriented, and it was agreed that only physically disabled residents would be admitted to the other homes. After one year the experiment was abandoned. The disoriented patient deteriorated even more rapidly in an atmosphere of total confusion. Patients who, in other settings, had made some attempt to be neat and to care for themselves gave up the ghost and allowed the staff to assume total responsibility for their care.

More dramatic was the turnover in personnel. The average length of employment was three months. The organization was unable to retain in a supervisory capacity even seasoned matrons with psychiatric training. When the facility was converted to general care and some of the residents were admitted to other homes in the group, staff morale and the attitudes of many of the patients improved. Not all the patients immediately became neat and untroublesome, but general improvement was exhibited in the mental attitudes of many.

Over the years I have found that frequently a mentally alert but physically handicapped patient will assume responsibility or a protective attitude toward a confused or untidy patient. Therefore, I do not feel we should, as a general rule, segregate the alert and confused resident. Naturally, if a patient becomes dangerous to himself or others, arrangements should be made for transfer to a more protective setting.

Regardless of the physical or mental status of your patients, if you expect them to enjoy living in your facility you must make it cheerful and comfortable for them. Warm, lively colors, cheerful drapes, and comfortable furnishings will make patients feel more at home. The careful grooming of your residents has a great effect on the general environment of your facility. As many patients as possible should be out of bed and dressed, their hair should be well groomed, the men should be shaved daily, attention should be paid to care of fingernails, eyeglasses, dentures, and ears. Some patients can perform these services for themselves and need only to be reminded to do so; others must have all the services performed for them. Think how much better a person looks and feels out of bed, dressed, and participating in activities with other patients. And, speaking of activities, during the past five years we have found programmed activities a part of all good nursing homes. The program must be limited to patient capabilities, but you'll be astonished how much can be done once you begin on an organized basis.

Community volunteers can be used as part of your activity program. Most groups visit your home at Christmas but would be happy to serve at other times if they knew they were welcome and the extent of the services you wished. However, beware of trying to use volunteers without someone to orient them as to your facility and to supervise them on a continuing basis.

When we speak of creating a favorable environment in a nursing home too often we think only of the patient-centered areas. What about a favorable working environment which will help the staff work more efficiently and comfortably? Any staff is bound to consider a good working climate as a highly desirable fringe benefit. A fair wage and worthy status are also basic. It makes a great deal of difference whether you call your staff members cleaners or housekeepers, attendants or aides. Do your employees have the opportunity to learn new skills; to advance to a better paying position or one with higher responsibility? Are you consistent about your rules, regulations, and requirements? Do you schedule work hours, work loads, holiday time impartially? Are you considerate of the feelings of your staff? Do you thank them for some minor service outside their realm of responsibility? Are you always accessible and approachable? Have you provided a place where staff may take their meals and/or their coffee break? Have you provided all the work-saving tools that make a job easier to do and are these tools in good repair?

If you are able to answer "yes" to all these questions, you have little turnover in personnel and are an expert in personnel relations. However, most of us tend to forget the staff and their needs, especially if they have been with us for a long time. What happens then is that working for you becomes "just a job" and many people stay on because it is easier than finding new employment. When this attitude prevails patient care becomes routine and patient feelings secondary. This can be the first breakdown in good patient care.

PATIENT CARE PROCEDURES

Good physical care is good business. Your reputation depends on how your patients are cared for, how they look, and how they smell. In order to be positive that each patient always looks fresh and neat, you must have a system. As we mentioned earlier, it is very important that every home should have a patient care plan. Some patients require a daily complete change in clothing to control odor; others may need a twice weekly change. Most older, sick patients require a daily bath, both to help control odor and to promote a feeling of well-being. The nursing staff should include routine mouth and denture care as part of their A.M. and P.M. service. At that time part of their observation should have to do with condition of the mouth and teeth. If a patient has any abnormalities they should be reported to the charge nurse who should call them to the attention of the physician. There should be a schedule for regular foot care, either by a visiting podiatrist or a member of the staff. There should also be a regular routine for shampoos and permanents.

Appearance of Patient

Regardless whether the patient is ambulatory or bedridden, the appearance should be always neat and fresh. If bedridden, the bed linen should be free of food debris, the blankets stain-free and in good repair, the bedsides and bed ends free of sticky food substances. The bedside table should not harbor stale food, soiled glasses, or tissues. The buttons, zippers, or hooks on clothing of ambulatory patients should be properly closed; their eyeglasses clean and in good repair; their shoes shined and with whole shoelaces in them. And lastly, take a good look at the wheelchair or rocking chair used by certain patients. Is food embedded in the cracks and crevices? Such chairs should be washed down at least once weekly and oftener for the incontinent patient.

Risks of Bed Rest

The informed physician of today is aware that bed rest is not prescribed without positive indications for its necessity. Merely to state the nefarious effects of bed rest constitutes a formidable list. Pulmonary, cardiac, gastrointestinal, urinary, musculoskeletal, and other systems are all adversely affected. Some of the risks of bed rest, such as bronchopneumonia, have long been recognized. In a nursing home the greatest danger from prolonged bed rest is the decubitus ulcers which are in reality areas of pressure necrosis. The most usual areas over which they form are those located over bony prominences subjected to long periods of unrelieved pressure. The lack of relief of pressure may be because of the patient's inability to move due to paralysis, or to the patient's additional inability to perceive discomfort due to loss of sensation. However, the formation of pressure areas in the nonparalyzed patient with good sensation is a common finding.

Prolonged immobilization complicates the picture by allowing a more rapid breakdown that interferes with healing. Maceration, due to soaking in urine and/or feces is another aggravating factor. Irregularities in the bedclothes, hard mattresses, and rough sheets are also not without importance in influencing the formation of these ulcerations. The prevention of decubitus ulcers consists principally of avoiding the above-mentioned causes. Cleanliness, dryness, and lack of pressure are the three cardinal principles in this avoidance. The maintenance of good protein balance is no doubt an additional important factor. In the severely ill patient, where immobilization cannot be avoided, such as in the case of an intertrochanteric fracture, or paraplegia due to spine fracture, continued immobilization in one position must be avoided at all costs. Frequent turning to allow recovery from short periods of pressure is essential. Other techniques may be profitably used, such as the Stryker or Bradford frame or the newer alternating pressure mattress.

Once decubitus ulcers have formed, their treatment follows the same principles as their prophylaxis—cleanliness, dryness, and lack of pressure. Ointments and salves are of little value. Where ulcerations are clean and shallow, the use of ultraviolet radiation with protection to surrounding skin can be useful. Where ulcerations are deep, healing can be very slow and, frequently, surgical closing may be necessary. Nursing staffs have been most ingenious in devising methods for treatment of decubitus ulcers. Some are without harm and where applied enthusiastically by the nursing staff, can really lead to the healing of the ulceration.

Attempts should be made to get each patient out of bed for at least one hour daily. In a few cases this may be impossible. Upon return to bed of the limited activity patient, the nursing staff should be aware of the following general principles:

Have the body in good alignment; try to approximate the same position as when the patient is standing.

Use a footboard to guard against foot drop.

Be sure the board is padded and has an extension block which prevents the mattress from touching it to prevent heel sores.

Do not keep patient's knees flexed for any great length of time. Often a nurse will catch the lower part of the bed to prevent the patient from sliding down in bed. This only increases the pressure on the calf and the heel; promotes venostasis of the lower extremities; and gives rise to thrombophlebitis.

Guard against external rotation of the hips which can throw the body out of alignment. The use of a trochanter roll can prevent this. This device can be made simply by using a rolled sheet about one inch thick and placing it between the patient's legs or under the lumbar sacral area.

Air rings frequently are used in nursing homes. However, you must be sure to underinflate them or you will decrease the circulation.

Very few bedfast patients do without a pillow on the bed. If pillows are employed they should also lift the shoulders in order not to shift the cervical spine forward and produce contractures. It is not uncommon to see the bed patient adopt a position in which the shoulders are internally rotated and elbows flexed. If maintained in this position for any length of time, or if this position is exaggerated by use of pillows, fixed deformities can result.

It is preferable to get a bed patient out and onto a commode, rather than allow him to use a bedpan. Studies indicate that use of a bedpan requires expenditure of more energy than use of a commode.

Physical Therapy

A large percentage of the patients admitted to nursing homes have a primary diagnosis of hemiplegia, characterized by muscle weakness of the involved upper and lower extremities, varying from slight to complete; increased spasticity, varying from slight to severe; aphasia, involving loss in communication by speaking, writing, etc.; impairment of memory orientation; and a deformity, involving the maintenance of a joint in a position other than the normal resting or functional position.

The nursing home's primary goals with such patients are to minimize the functional loss by preventing complications of deformity; to prevent decubitus ulcers and depression; and to help patients achieve independent ambulation, self-care and adequate communication. For example, spasticity in a lower leg interferes with voluntary function but this may be controlled by means of a leg brace; aphasia, which may interfere with communication and understanding, often yields to consistent retraining effort; and incontinence may be relieved as a part of the patient's general improvement.

For such patients as these the services of a trained physical therapist are invaluable. We do not mean to imply that every nursing home should have a therapist on its staff, nor that each patient must be visited daily by a therapist. However, under the supervision of a physician, the patient should be evaluated as to rehabilitation potential by a therapist. Therapy techniques should be instituted by the therapist and staff members should be trained in these techniques, so that any gains realized may be maintained. The services of a registered physical therapist may be purchased from a community agency or hospital or, in some metropolitan areas, may be shared by a group of nursing homes. Your real goal is to help the patient toward increased independence in self-care, which will mean a lessened need for professional nursing care.

Where a therapist is not available, or if for some reason it is not feasible to use one, staff members should be oriented in methods to help the hemiplegic patient attain maximum self-care. Some of the simple procedures are: to encourage as much use as possible of the nonaffected hand; to encourage use of the affected arm as an assistive device; to teach activities that require use of only one arm; to encourage bearing weight on the affected leg, or obtain a leg brace and train the patient in putting it on and taking it off; and to teach transfer activities and ambulation.

Such a patient may be taught how to dress through the use of front-opening clothing with zippers; by learning to place the affected leg into a garment first and remove it last; by using the normal arm to pull an affected leg through openings; by wearing slip-on shoes, or putting elastic shoelaces into shoes. He may be taught how to shower by use of a stool and grab bar; to care for his teeth and to shave himself by learning methods of one-hand squeezing of tooth paste and shaving cream; how to use a long handled sponge to wash affected parts; and how to stabilize articles which ordinarily call for the use of two hands. These procedures, when used after careful evaluation of the patient in terms of individual and social needs, often directly aid in increasing the level of function. While they rarely return a person to active employment, they do add to his own self-esteem.

Religious Practices

Every patient in a nursing home should be allowed visitation by the pastor of his choice. This is particularly important to a patient in a critical phase, and is considered essential for Catholic patients. Do not wait until the patient is comatose before calling the clergyman. This may serve to allay your own feelings, but it accomplishes little for the patient. To the Catholic patient the last rites have essential meaning.

Prior to the visit of the priest, prepare a table near the patient's bedside with a crucifix, two blessed candles, several small balls of cotton, a glass of water, and a spoon. Loosen the bedclothes around the patient's feet and place the hands outside the blanket. When the priest arrives, light the candles and ask whether he wishes you to remain and assist him. In most cases the priest realizes how busy things are and is quite willing to turn back the bedclothing and anoint the feet and hands himself and to give the patient a sip of water after receiving communion. In the event a patient dies prior to a priest's being called, notify the proper church and you will be instructed what to do.

Talking with the various pastors who visit your nursing home and finding out their preference with regard to final visitation, will enable you to make a note of each denomination's procedures in your procedure manual.

Administrators and owners of nursing homes, public, private and voluntary, are in an unenviable position. Most of them are conscientious people, and some are truly dedicated. For many, the job entails hard physical work and emotional strain. For most the monetary rewards are small. The satisfactions of achievement may be limited by the fact that, in spite of the best that can be done for them, many patients cannot be changed in body or mind. Nursing home administrators are subject to many pressures. On the one hand, they can see the need for physical improvement in their plants, better qualified staff, and additional ancillary services to their residents. On the other hand, they are faced with the fact that most people who need nursing home care have limited funds with which to pay for it. Even government insurance benefits are limited. Administrators may endorse improvement in quality of care, only to be faced with the reality that such improvements must be accompanied by a rise in rates which may preclude care to those most in need of it.

Undeniably, a more concerted effort is needed by nursing home administrators and owners, as a group, to make the public aware of the services rendered in these facilities.

Chapter 5

The Administrator's Relationship to Patient Care

MARGIE S. DAVIS, *R.N.*

Types of residents to be admitted to nursing homes are usually determined by state regulations or by state statutes, and then further decided by individual health establishments. Such facilities may not be permitted to care for persons with communicable diseases, including active tuberculosis; pregnancy—one week before and one week after delivery; alcoholism—chronic compulsive types; treatment of children fifteen years of age or younger; persons who have been diagnosed or adjudged to have acute psychotic conditions, or who are dangerous to themselves or to others.

The health care facility may choose to specialize in the care of cerebral vascular accident cases, fractures, diabetics, cancer patients, etc. This information should certainly be included in a facility's brochure. The admission agreement should fix the responsibility for carrying it out. Admission records should be kept and a definite policy should provide for arranging admissions of patients. Patients may or may not make their own arrangements for admission to the home, depending upon their mental and physical condition. Responsibility for payments and decisions must definitely be established. The responsible family member, friend, or conservator should be designated, as well as the third-party involvement of state agencies or voluntary health insurance companies.

RELATIONSHIPS WITH FAMILY AND VISITORS

Although most of you have brochures covering many types of information, the initial contact with families is usually made over the telephone. The telephone is the home's best public relations tool. And the administrator or receptionist must never be too busy to answer telephone inquiries. If you do not have a vacancy, you should help the person find one.

If the family has been pleased and impressed by the telephone conversation, the next step will be a visit to see the home and meet the owners and/or administrator. The family may or may not bring the patient to see the facility.

The administrator must relieve the family of all guilt or stigma. This is especially true if the physical condition is accompanied by a mental condition. The family often subconsciously rejects the patient, and at the same time may be torn between a duty to care for the old person and the sacrifice to self and neglect of other members of the family. Listen and sympathize with the family and convince them they are doing the right thing in placing their loved one where he or she will have professional care and be able to socialize with people of his own era, since often the past becomes more important to such persons than the present or future.

Services of the Home

Your services are for sale. If you sell these services thoroughly and completely to families and visitors, your problems will be minimal. Although you have a brochure explaining your services, policies, and procedures, take time to explain this during the initial interview. Let them see the physical plant; show them your home environment and point out how it differs from that of a hospital. Show them your menus, and explain to them the importance of regular, balanced meals. Show them the orderliness, cleanliness, and efficiency of your administration as reflected in the condition of your guests. Encourage them to talk with your nurses or patients. Protect yourself against the inaccurate description of the patient's condition by his family. You must know the patient's condition—physical and mental and his degree of body control.

Take time to visit, if only for a few minutes, with relatives and visitors. Strive for complete family confidence. By placing their loved one with you, a seed of confidence has already been planted. Permit visiting at all hours, day or night. This dispels any doubt that you are trying to deceive them. Invite relatives in at mealtime to see their relative's tray, or to be your guest for lunch. This certainly eliminates all fear about your food.

Good service is the secret of the successful home. Always follow the wishes of the patient, considering his needs, likes and dislikes as far as possible. Keep families informed about the patient's condition at all times. Be frank about the patient's sleeping, eating, and personal habits. If the patient is untidy, and it is impossible to keep him clean and dry, it is much better for you to discuss this condition with the family beforehand than to have them find out on their own.

The home administrator must be all things to all people. This includes the family. You may be caught in the middle of family situations where children haven't even spoken in years. Your duty is to get them to put the patient first. It is not unusual that a family may require more of the administrator's and staff's time than the actual time needed to care for the patient. Family cooperation is needed in planning for the patient. Oldsters, like children, may be overprotected or neglected, and usually resent being told what to do by their children. Enforce compliance with your policies regarding your home. These policies must not be verbal but written. This helps to gain acceptance because obviously they are intended for all.

Service by the Family

Family interest may be stimulated in the patient by permitting visiting hours at the family's convenience. Encourage the giving of useful gifts and the bringing of food, if approved by the administrator. Encourage parties, overnight visits with the family, birthday recognition, and celebrating such special occasions as Christmas, Easter, etc. The family may do the personal laundry, help with personal hygiene, or may be invited to come at mealtime and help feed the patient. The family can also help with walks, rides, taking the patient to church, or help with a church service in the home. In order to have maximum visiting, it is my firm belief that an open-door policy is by far the best method, permitting visiting over the 24-hour day. If you limit visiting, do it gracefully, and provide a suitable place with maximum privacy.

We have found it helpful to substitute or supplement family visiting with visits from volunteer organizations—Red Cross, Gray Ladies, Scouts, lodges, and local church groups. These visits may be combined with lectures, movies, or parties in the home. You may wish to regulate entrances and exits by designating the specific entrance and exit. Visitors should be announced. You may wish to control visitors who have colds, have been drinking, or perhaps a family member who is upsetting or depressing to the patient. It has been my experience that frequent short visits are more helpful to the patient than long infrequent ones.

Never discuss the patient's condition with a visitor. The condition of a patient (especially the aphasic patient) should never be discussed in his presence by anyone. Protect yourself against false reports by patients to relatives or visitors. Although a relative or visitor may realize that illness has affected his capacity for mental precision, lifelong habits of trusting and believing him may be even stronger.

PATIENT ADMISSIONS

When the patient is admitted there should be a thorough check, and admission notes should include general appearance, nutrition, skin condition, abrasions, etc. Temperature, pulse, and respiration readings should be taken, as well as the blood pressure. The TPR and BP may be repeated on each shift for five days to establish a norm for the patient. Discretion should be used in regard to an admission bath. Clothes and personal possessions should be marked and an inventory made. Valuables should be noted, and if left in the patient's possession, the administrator should have a signed statement of release from responsibility for the items which the patient or family insists on his keeping under his own control.

The administrator or admitting personnel should make all information learned during interview and admission available to the staff. For example, a brief social history of the patient and family may be included on the back of your record.

Make your new resident feel at home. A tour with introductions to other residents is a good method; radiate friendliness, cheerfulness, and readiness to please. Smile and be a good listener. Welcome and discuss complaints. If the emotional reactions or other demands of a patient prove to be beyond what you can ever hope to satisfy, then frankly suggest that another home might better fill his need.

PATIENT DISCHARGE OR TRANSFER

The patient's physician is responsible for the discharge of patients to their families, or transfer of patients to hospitals or other homes. The resident should be released upon the attending physician's orders to the person placing him in your home. A home cannot prevent a resident's leaving, unless he has been declared incompetent and committed to your home by due process of law. Should the resident leave against your advice before someone comes for him, every attempt should be made to have him sign his own release, relieving the home of any responsibility for resulting injury. If the resident should refuse to sign the release, witnesses should be called in to observe the advice being giving regarding possible injury. The witness should sign a statement (to become a part of the patient's record), that he witnessed the events leading to the patient's leaving the home. The attending physician may leave written instructions with the administrator for medication and treatment to be continued with the patient at home. Reassure the family that if your services are needed again, the patient is welcome to return to your home. The family may need help in finding housekeeping services, or if nursing is going to be needed, you may want to refer them to the local Visiting Nurse Service.

If the transfer is to a hospital, much apprehension may be dispelled by assuring the patient that his stay is only temporary. A copy of the patient's orders should accompany him, along with a brief history of the signs and symptoms of his present condition. In the case of a fall or accident, explicit details should be given. This same courtesy should be extended by the hospital when the resident returns to the home.

If your patient is transferred to a nursing home from a boarding home, a certain amount of emotional conditioning or preparation is needed to make it acceptable. The transfer from one nursing home to another nursing home may be just as upsetting to the patient since he has become adjusted where he is and doesn't want to start a new life. When patients are transferred from one nursing home to another, copies of the current medication and treatment should be sent to the nursing home, along with refunds, if any, and other pertinent information.

HOME-HOSPITAL RELATIONSHIPS

For all your hospital contacts, be very sure to consult the hospital administrator first and obtain his permission for any other contacts you may wish to make. Visit the hospital frequently. Invite key personnel to visit your home. Snapshot brochures in the hands of doctors, nurses, social workers, receptionists, etc., may help your home get hospital referrals. Hospitals should not be your competitors; they should be your co-workers rendering a different kind of service. If a nursing home-hospital affiliation is desired, plans and procedures should be worked out in advance of need. A close liaison with the social service department in the hospital in dealing with old age assistance cases is a must. For a formal, prepared nursing home-hospital relationship, I refer you to the Illinois or Colorado Hospital Associations. For a list called Hospital-Nursing Home Relationships, I refer you to the United States Department of Health, Education and Welfare, Public Health Service, Division of Hospital and Medical Facilities, Program Evaluation and Reports Branch, Washington 25, D.C.

In a system where homes have their own organized medical staff, with provision for emergency medical service, it is proposed that the physicians privileged to treat patients be organized into an active and associate staff. The administrator of the home, along with the medical staff, should develop rules and regulations covering the qualifications for admission to the staff, as well as evaluating criteria for acceptance of the staff. The medical staff in turn should adopt policies, with the approval of the administration, to govern their professional work. Model constitutions and by-laws for hospital medical staffs may be obtained from the American Hospital Association, 850 North Lakeshore Drive, Chicago 11, Illinois.

The homes may provide optional "house physician" services to their residents. This may be desirable, where financial resources are low. (This has been very satisfactory in the state of Oregon where doctors were assigned to X numbers of patients in X numbers of nursing homes.) This arrangement assures you a physician whom you know well, can trust, and with whom you can discuss each patient's problems as they arise. This also gives you a medical resource to call on for planning patient care, or for any medical administrative problems. Several factors should be considered when selecting a "house physician." Look for interest and understanding of the aged. You will find that some physicians are more interested in the aged than are others.

Until a few short years ago, there was no recognition of geriatrics or gerontology in courses in medical schools. Not only is gerontology a part of many medical schools today, but workshops in this area are also being held for practicing physicans. Be sure the physician knows your home, the services you have to offer, and also your limitations. Does he know that you are not a hospital? Select a physician willing to come to your home day and night when a patient is near death, or in other types of emergencies. The physician must have available time to talk to the patient after his examination. Five minutes of the physician's time can do more for the patient than five hours of the administrator's time. Know your physician well, see him in action before you choose your "house physician."

Where a home requires residents to designate their physicians, it permits them to cooperate with all doctors who send their patients, and it also respects each patient's choice of his own personal physician. If the patient or family asks you to suggest a doctor, always suggest two or more, thus letting the patient or his family make the final decision. Your medical society may have a liaison committee for this purpose. Don't play favorites; instead, work with all of them.

Recognize the doctor as an expert. His word is final and he takes the responsibility for being right. He is not, however, an expert in nursing home or home for aged administration. Deal ethically with the doctor, build up the patient's confidence in him and always understand his orders. Should you not understand certain medical terminology, or how to spell the name of some medication, ask questions. The doctor will welcome them. Carry out his orders promptly, correctly, and conscientiously. The administrator's attitude toward the doctor sets the pattern for the home and the entire staff. Call the physician only when necessary and inform him correctly about the patient's condition. Your system of record-keeping will make the patient's current condition readily available to your physician. When I hear a nursing home administrator say, "I can't get my doctors to write on my charts," it is time then, I think, for him to evaluate his relationship with his doctors.

POLICIES AND PROCEDURES

Since written nursing procedures are a must in any facility where nursing care is given, the following procedure guides will be found very helpful: *Basic Nursing,* Gill, Helen Z., R.N., The Macmillan Co., N.Y., 1957; *How to be a Nursing Aide in a Nursing Home,* American Nursing Home Association, 1346 Connecticut Avenue, N.W., Washington 6, D.C.; *Practical Nursing Today, Attitudes, Knowledge, Skills,* Kelly, Cordelia W., G. P. Putnam's Sons, 1958.

Your policies regarding working hours, schedules, and case loads will be partially decided for you by state laws which have been designed to protect the employee. Many matters of policy are, of course, the prerogative of the administrator. For example, he has the right to require all employees to sign in and sign out. This can be done by using a time book or a time clock. It is just as important for an employee to leave work on time as it is for him to arrive on time. Rest periods and meal periods are legally required. Split shifts may present a problem, because of meals and the span of time of the shift. An excellent way to provide the staff at the needed time is to hire two people for 4-hour shifts. The value of part-time employees should not be overlooked, especially in regard to paying overtime. Should an employee on a three- or four-day week need to work an extra day, the employer will not have to pay overtime.

Every attempt should be made to adjust the work load properly, so that one employee will not be standing around while another is under pressure to perform his tasks. Only by writing of specific work directions for a large number of tasks can the administrator solve the confusion of nursing home administration. The answer to this is job analysis, or job specifications for each employee in your home. If you know the work of each shift, and if you obtain the help of each person on each shift, your job analysis can soon be done. Simply have each person, for a period of time, write down every five minutes what he was doing. After a comparative analysis of these results, you will know much more precisely what kinds of work you are scheduling. A simple way to do work schedules is to arrange tasks by the clock and also arrange employee work hours by the clock. The work schedule must vary in order to cover each day, as the daily schedules may vary.

Another consideration in making schedules is getting the patients and employees matched as to personalities. Generally the older person does better with the same nurse and fewer changes in his routine. After the total volume of work is assorted and assigned to certain hours on certain days, one must still divide the work among individuals and get each individual to carry his part of the load. This can be done only with constant supervision, which will insure that the work is distributed properly, and all assigned tasks are completed. The rotating of shifts or duties may be used to determine the work output. The time required by different individuals to perform the same tasks can be used as a guideline for performance.

It is also in order for the administrator to ask: Are coffee breaks and smoking time abused? Is there a misuse of time for personal telephone calls? These are but a few of the factors which enter into the production of the individual employee.

I would say that written policies are essential to good nursing home administration. We have already discussed the need for written admission, transfer, and discharge policies. There should also be a printed statement as to the kind of residents that are to be admitted, their economic level, requirements for care, level of mental competence, etc. For example, there should be answers to such questions as: Are seniles acceptable? Are family status, religious affiliation, medical supervision, and nursing care considerations?

Your employment and personnel policies should include such matters as: who will be employed, health requirements (usually set by the rules and regulations of a state statute), and conditions of employment. Most manuals of nursing care routine (I recommend our *Manual for the Operation of a Small Nursing Home,* published by the Colorado Nursing Home Association) discuss these and numerous other details with which nursing home personnel should be thoroughly familiar.

NURSING AND PERSONNEL SERVICES

Your supervisory nursing personnel (registered nurses) should have experience, if possible, with the aged and chronically ill patient. The duties of the licensed practical nurse are usually outlined by law in each state where there is a Nurse Practice Act. Her duties may overlap with the duties of the nurse aide, depending upon the number of personnel and the type of patients. The nurse aide does not administer medication nor give treatments. The orderly assists the nurses and aides with heavy work and gives some treatment to male patients.

STERILIZATION FACILITIES

A room or designated area in the nursing home, away from the kitchen or other food preparation area, should be used to clean and sterilize nursing supplies and equipment. Water should completely cover the objects to be sterilized and these should be boiled for 20 minutes to destroy spore-forming organisms. A strainer-covered container should be provided for surgical asepsis. Catheters should be sterilized. Dishes, bedpans, and urinals should be sterilized by steam. The autoclave used for enema equipment should be steamed under pressure. Trays with catheterizers, surgical dressings, or irrigators should be set up using a double muslin wrapper. These trays may be stored for only a week to 10 days, then they must be reautoclaved. Chemicals may be used for sterilization.

ADMINISTRATON OF DRUGS

The administration of drugs and oxygen is a grave responsibility and every precaution should be taken to eliminate the possibility of errors. A definite plan for the administration of drugs should be set up by the nursing home. These are described in our Colorado manual, as follows:

1. Read the order for medication carefully from the medicine card (sheet, book).
2. Read the label three (3) times. (Never use unmarked containers.)
3. Always identify a medication by its name instead of *Rx* number.
4. Know your patient and be sure he's taking his medication.
5. All medications must be taken in the nurse's presence.
6. The nurse who prepares the medication should administer same.
7. Keep medicine cabinet locked at all times.
8. Never put liquid medicine back into the bottles. Pills may be replaced if dry and untouched.
9. A schedule for medications should be set up—9-1-5, 10-2-6, 8-12-4. After set up, adhere to schedule.
10. Never attempt to give medication by mouth to a patient who cannot swallow or who is semiconscious (new CVA cases).
11. If a mistake is made in measuring and giving a medication, report it immediately to the person in charge.

You may wish to post a list of medical abbreviations and clinical weights and measures, since not all your staff may be familiar with these.

CONTROL OF NARCOTICS AND OTHER DRUGS

1. A medication should be stored in a locked cabinet.
2. Special precaution should be taken with drugs marked "poison."
3. Individual patient containers can be easily made from plastic sherbet containers, metal bread trays.
4. If the nursing home keeps narcotics on hand, a permit from the Federal Bureau of Narcotics must be obtained. Special records must then be kept: name of patient, date, time of administration, and names of prescribing physicians.
5. Homes not having a narcotic permit, and where each patient has his own physician who prescribes the narcotics, must, upon discharge or death of the patient, return all unused narcotics to the Federal Bureau of Narcotics. (In some states the Health Department will return them, and usually your pharmacist will handle this for you.)

OXYGEN THERAPY

Oxygen should be administered only when ordered by the doctor, and no one should attempt to administer oxygen unless he has had the appropriate training. The tent and nasal catheter are the two methods most often used in nursing homes. Safety precautions should include: private room, if possible; no smoking signs; no visitors; the securing of the cylinder, so it cannot be pushed over; and opening of the cylinder before attaching regulator. Do not use oil or alcohol as back rubs on patients under oxygen. Do not use oil or grease on regulators and always store cylinders in a cool, dry place away from sparks, grease, radiators, and paint, and again secure cylinders to the wall by chain or rope.

LABORATORY SERVICES

Laboratory services may be procured either through the nursing home-hospital agreement, or, if you are in a metropolitan area, private laboratories and even portable X-ray units are available to serve your patients. Only in very large facilities is it feasible for nursing homes to have their own laboratories.

RESIDENT'S ENVIRONMENT

I like the statement, "A nursing home is the shadow of the administrator." In many states the major emphasis has been placed on the physical aspects of buildings and equipment. Although these criteria may conceivably make for efficient operation, they are not sufficient to insure the best possible care of patients. I take issue with the statement that private and semiprivate rooms are more desirable than wards. One may eliminate friction, but to leave the oldster in a private room to continue the vegetative process is not always desirable. This, again, will depend largely upon the type of patients in your home. The basic equipment in the home is usually delineated by the state standards. The homelike atmosphere is desirable in nursing homes and homes for the aged. We are not hospitals and should not try to look like them.

HYGIENE OF THE AGED PATIENT

I shall not go into the physical changes and effects of the aging process. You, as administrators, already have some knowledge of these factors. However, I would say that every home should develop policies regarding the frequency of baths, care of hands, feet, oral hygiene, bed positioning, housekeeping, safety measures, etc. These are among the procedures which should be written up as part of the policies of the home.

An attempt at a written statement, dealing with patient care to insure comfort, prevent bedsores, and enhance nutrition, might be as follows:

Patients who cannot change their own positions should be changed at least every two hours. Proper positioning is important—footboards and sandbags should be employed as well as back, face, and side positions. Feet can be elevated with discretion in the event of hip flexion contractures.

Sitting should be out of bed, unless written orders are given for the patient to remain in bed continuously.

There should be positioning of hand and forearm for paralytics, hemiplegics, or paraplegics.

The chief causes of decubitus ulcers are dehydration, malnutrition, and impaired circulation, in conjunction with poor skin care. If skin care techniques are improved, tissues will heal almost spontaneously. If malnutrition or dehydration causes the ulcer, the healing process is much longer, of course.

"An ounce of prevention is worth a pound of cure," is certainly true in preventing decubitus ulcers. First toilet train your patient as you would an ordinary two-year-old. This can be done, unless the patient has retention of urine or is a "dribbler." Keep the patient as dry as possible. Wash with soap and water every two hours if the patient is a dribbler.

While cleaning the ulcer, gently massage even to the point that bright red blood may appear near the edges. Get the patient out of bed and, if unable to do this, at least change his position every two hours.

Supplemental feedings of Gevral protein or other forms of concentrated protein should be given. Put the patient on intake and output, to remind your staff to force fluids. (An incontinent patient with an indwelling Foley catheter can have the catheter irrigated without ever changing the patient's position. This fact is one of the reasons why I prefer to care for the aged without catheters.)

Caution should be used in applying benzoin and other medication to toughen the skin. These should only be used if ordered by the physician.

First consult the attending physician for the prescribed treatment. However, a correction of the causes will start the healing process immediately. White cotton anklets make an excellent protective covering for ankles and heels.

Never limit fluids to an incontinent patient. Instead, force fluids. Only a small percentage of incontinency is caused by illness or disease. In a majority of cases incontinency is caused by psychological factors. Toilet train your patient. Change the patient's position every two hours. Get him up in a chair two or three times daily.

An airfoam mattress may be used, or sheepskin sawdust mattress, to distribute pressure areas. Eliminate wrinkles in the undersheets, force fluids, increase the protein intake, and apply gentle massage to the ulcers.

If prescribed by the physician, infra-red treatment is wonderful to stimulate healing and help keep the area dry.

EMERGENCIES

Provision should be made for the efficient handling of emergencies in the home. Written policies and procedures should be developed, approved by your attending physician and posted at each nurse's station. Some of the conditions might be as follows: bruises, cuts, fractures, nosebleeds, fainting, fractures, heart attacks, cerebral vascular accidents.

Every home should, with the help of a physician, establish a standard for supplies to be kept on hand. The first-aid kit or emergency tray should include tourniquet, bandages, dressings, adhesive tape, alcohol, merthiolate, stimulants, caramine, Metrazole, sterile syringes (2-10-50 cc size), hypodermic and intravenous needles, 50 cc of 50 per cent glucose, or the new medicine for diabetics (which may be given orally).

The telephone numbers of the police department, fire department, ambulances, hospitals, taxis, and pharmacies should be posted at each phone throughout the building.

POLICIES OF RELIGIOUS GROUPS

The majority of Protestant patients will appreciate having their ministers notified when they are admitted to your home, or are critically ill. Christian Scientists believe illness can be cured by faith. The Seventh Day Adventists worship on Saturday instead of Sunday. They follow very closely certain regulations found in the Old Testament, including not eating meats forbidden in the Book of Leviticus. Some very strict observers eat no meat at all. Jehovah's Witnesses will not allow a transfusion of blood to be given. Mormons do not, as a rule, take any stimulants—coffee, tea, etc. A priest should be notified when the Catholic patient is admitted, or in critical condition.

In the case of a Catholic patient, the nurse should be familiar with the following sacraments, as it may be necessary for her to assist the priest, at some points.

1. Baptism—usually performed by the priest, but may be done by any who will perform it in the prescribed way—water poured on the forehead, while the person says aloud: "I baptize thee in the name of the Father, and the Son and the Holy Ghost." If it is unknown whether he has been baptized before, the formula is said conditionally, "If thou are *not* previously baptized. . . ."

2. Confession, with complete privacy, is heard by a priest who, through Christ, has the power to forgive sins.

3. Holy Eucharist (Holy Communion) may be brought to the sick. When no emergency exists, certain preparation is made. Cover the bedside table with a white cloth. A glass of water, a spoon, a crucifix, two candles, and matches are placed thereon. Communion given to the dying is called Holy Visticum.

4. Extreme Unction (Last Rites) is reserved for those in danger of death from sickness or after an accident. If there is time, the patient is prepared as for Holy Communion. In addition, a small piece of cotton is provided. The bedclothes should be loosened so that the feet can be anointed. Whenever possible, the priest should be notified of a dying patient's need for his services before the patient loses consciousness.

The nurse should be alert to sacred articles in or around the patient's bed. Care should be taken to remove rosary beads and other medals attached to the patient's gown before it is put in the laundry. The Catholic patient is obligated to attend Mass on Sunday and Holy Days, to abstain from eating flesh meat on Friday, and to fast during Lent and other prescribed days. This obligation is not binding if the health of the patient is likely to be impaired.

The three major groups within the Jewish faith are Orthodox, Conservative, and Reformed. The Orthodox Jew adheres to strict dietary regulations and customs. In the home, one set of dishes is used for meat and another for milk products. A rabbi should be called when a Jewish patient is critically ill. Nothing is done to the body following death, except to change soiled dressings. The mortuary should be notified in advance, if possible, since they have to remove the body from the home immediately. Burial is arranged the following day in a Jewish cemetery, unless the death occurs on Friday, when the body must be buried before sundown. Burials are not permitted on Saturday, the Jewish Sabbath.

Chapter 6

Care of Disabled Residents

ISABEL MacRAE, *R.N., M.A.*

Two major objectives should be kept in mind in the care of disabled residents of nursing and retirement homes: first, optimum function for the individual within the limits of his capacity, and second, the enlargement of the limits of that capacity. These objectives, faithfully adhered to, will make for independence in activities of daily living and the widening of physical and social horizons.

I have selected six words, a discussion of which will, I believe, help to make clear our rehabilitative task with disabled elderly residents. The words are: Prevention, Persistence, Personalization, Potential, Process, and Procedure. These might be called the "Six Promising P's." Let us, then, start with *Prevention.*

PREVENTION

Of course, it is our hope that from the earliest indication of debility every effort will be made to help the patient to prevent further development of his disability or dysfunction. Too often we find that because of ignorance, lack of interest, or inability, the preventive measures are not initiated. But this need not preclude the effort now to prevent further disability, and this we can institute. There are many aspects of prevention. We know, for instance, that muscles not active become incapable of activity; one may note a recently admitted bed patient—hemiplegic or arthritic—remaining curled up on his side most of the time. This will surely lead to joint contractures, especially of the hinge joints at knee and elbow. A twice-daily routine of range-of-motion exercises to all the joints, emphasizing extension of the joint, will at least prevent further deterioration and should reduce whatever contracture tendency is established. To remain in one position for long periods also threatens the integrity of the skin—pressure sores are, after all, caused by pressure.

Prevention of further disability, then, requiries establishment of a regular routine of position change and stimulation of circulation to every pressure point—shoulder, elbow, hip, knees, ankles, shoulder blades, coccyx, and sacrum. I am a strong advocate of the regular application of the flat of the hand to these areas on a routine basis. In addition, the skin must be kept resilient, dry, and well nourished. Thus, diet becomes a preventive measure and the person who has his dentures in will make best use of the protein foods with which he is provided. "Diet," for the average patient without cardiac or kidney disorders, must include adequate fluids, which means a total of two quarts daily, not all of it necessarily water. This schedule has definite, positive effects on both skin turgor and elimination habits. The higher the level of general physical well-being a person enjoys, the freer he is to turn his attention to something other than himself; and conversely, the more satisfying social stimulus the person receives, the less his interest will be centered upon his own bodily function. Social networks, when maintained or reestablished, do appear to lead to improved physical response by giving motivation for making physical effort.

PERSISTENCE

Every one of the other five "P's" depends, in some degree, for its success upon *Persistence*. Only by persistence can prevention of further or new disability be achieved; only by persistence can new objectives be reached. We all know that no single method works with every patient, and we know also that basically there is no "status quo" in relation to the living body; it is always in a state of establishing and reestablishing equilibrium. Patients who do not improve, regress; that is where motivation enters into the picture. Even those people who are grossly disabled can achieve wonderful improvement if they are properly guided and highly motivated to persist.

But how to motivate? Zane and Lowenthal[1] have identified motivation as a complex of forces; some are negative and some are positive. They conclude that when stress arises, negative factors become dominant; positive factors dominate with decreasing stress. In the clinical situation, stress arises when the person anticipates that he cannot achieve what he wishes to do—that is, anticipated failure increases stress. One aspect of rehabilitation, then, is to strengthen positive factors by providing goals which are possible for the individual to achieve and, through this, to change or improve his motivation. I am sure each of us has encountered the various kinds of poor motivation illustrated by the person who refuses to try; the one who gives up too easily; and the one who, apparently, cannot learn.

In handling these situations a variety of approaches is possible. I have already mentioned the breakdown of the goal into attainable parts. Perhaps the problem lies within the patient, unrecognized even by him: neurological or visual and perceptive defects may affect a person's performance, for example, in handling table utensils. Close analysis of the conditions in which the performer fails may reveal clues to the remedy and increase the positive factors in his motivation. The person who occupies his therapy time complaining about a variety of things cannot spend it in concentrated effort to improve function. If the worker will repeatedly recall the patient's attention to the task at hand, the complaints will be replaced, at least temporarily, by therapeutic effort and some degree of success.

In this area of motivation, the worker must be very careful not to make unsupported judgments or to be unappreciative of the effort made by the patient. The warmth and encouragement of the worker have a profound effect on the patient's desire to improve and thereby to please him; conversely, fear of the worker's disapproval sometimes immobilizes the patient and prevents his achieving as much as he is capable of doing. Poor motivation may be manifest by lack of involvement (lack of interest) in the whole project. This is often the initial response. Lacklustre performance and regression from previously satisfactory performance are other manifestations of poor motivation. But, rather than thinking about the motivation as such, it is usually more profitable for the therapist to think about the stress factors in the situation which may inhibit learning. Above all, rehabilitation is a process of relearning how to function adequately.

PERSONALIZATION

In speaking of motivation I have so far emphasized the plain hard work and therapist-patient relationship. But the next "P"—*Personalization*—includes many of motivation's positive factors. Man is a social being and as long as he is able to be independent in the activities of his daily life, he will reject the idea of himself as "old." He may be "elderly," but when he acknowledges that he is "old," he is also identifying the fact that his level of self-esteem is no longer as high as it has been previously.

The emphasis in our society upon the desirability of youth has unfortunately implied that age is undesirable. This area of self-esteem is the one in which greatest stress reactions to aging develop, and the person who is abruptly, and perhaps unexpectedly, retired usually demonstrates these reactions very clearly. The same abrupt assault to the image of the self as a capable, achieving, contributing individual occurs to the person, whatever his age, who suffers a heart attack or a cerebral vascular accident. And many persons resist admission to a nursing home because they resent the implication of being "on the shelf," where they no longer can contribute as before. But as long as it is possible to find some way in which the elderly in our care can continue their current, useful mechanisms for the preservation of self-esteem or to establish new ones, they will be motivated toward independence at their own optimum level. When self-care is given a high positive value, it becomes more desirable than being "waited on."

These mechanisms will vary in kind or emphasis, but the worker's persistence in the personalization effort pays big dividends. In speaking of motivation I suggested looking at the factors which caused the particular individual to anticipate failure. This is certainly one form of personalization. So is the utilization of all you learn in conversation with each person about his former home, the kinds of adjustments he found effective and satisfying, the kinds of social contacts he enjoyed, and so on. Knowing that a resident previously has been a member of many clubs, for example, will give a clue as to the response you might expect from him about social activity in the nursing home.

Group membership, however tenuous, appears to be necessary for healthy self-esteem. We all want to belong, and if you are alert for small signs of such a sense in your less sociable patients, they can be encouraged and the individual's social horizons and activities expanded. An incident reported by Landau[2] gives a good example of this: a man who frequently attended a Day Center, sitting in the same chair, but rarely conversing with anyone, was seen emptying ash trays one day as one of the workers was showing a new member around. The worker recognized this activity as an indication of the man's sense of belonging to the center, and she reinforced it by asking the man to help her to make the new member feel welcome. The man did so, with evident pleasure, and by enumerating the attractions of the Day Center he increased his own sense of involvement and worthiness. To fulfill acceptable social roles in the new setting will make the roles which have been relinquished less appealing and will maintain the person's self-esteem. But people need help to learn what, in this particular society, is approved. Every nursing or retirement home is its own small society, with its own set of acceptable and unacceptable behaviors which each new member must be helped to learn. Because each new member has his unique pattern of response to social stimuli, one must again be wary of making unsubstantiated judgments.

POTENTIAL

Closely allied with Personalization is *Potential;* for how can one individualize his care of a person without gaining clues as to the potential of that person? Our judgments about the learning capacity of elderly people rest on questionable evidence (mostly I.Q. tests, which are concerned with areas we find easy to measure, but which are not necessarily where the greatest strengths of the elderly lie). We know that the elderly maintain their language skills and that these are involved in all intellectual activities. We know also that learning is burdensome only when other goals are more attractive, as playing is to school children.

If a man wants to improve his garden or a woman wants to gain a reputation as the best breadmaker in town, each of them finds the learning involved no burden. If we can make the process a creative one, learning, in this case how to achieve independence in daily living, will be more attractive. This is one of the big advantages which occupational therapy has over physical therapy. While each is aimed at restoration of function, the latter is undisguised hard work, and the former includes a large element of creativity. Social activities enjoy the same advantage. They are enjoyable to the participants and, at the same time, increase motivation toward further participation. This adds greatly to the patient's sense of independence. Creativity increases the positive factors in motivation to achieve. Accomplishment improves self-esteem; and this, in turn, increases freedom to participate in learning, with the expectation of success. The old saying that "nothing succeeds like success" may be a questionable cliché in some educative processes, but it is invariably an appropriate expression in rehabilitative effort.

Not only do the persons involved have potential, but there is potential in every situation. When existence is monotonous, apathy and depression, perhaps even mental deterioration and disorientation, ensue. Since we know that every nursing home has more than enough for its staff members to do, it may well be that a change of emphasis is in order. I am convinced that a shift in major emphasis from "care" to more stimulation of the residents to learn to care for themselves is in order. The satisfactions derived from this change in approach would be shared by both residents and staff.

No one underrates the amount of effort and time required by rehabilitative procedures, but no one who has seen the results will underestimate the value of them. Kelman[3] suggests that activities designed to stimulate, motivate, and aid disabled residents in using their capacities for self-care may well be more important than restorative programs. I am sure they are more attractive to residents. Group activities do many things. Contact with others is a prime source of restored self-esteem, as I have already indicated. This leads to involvement with the group; involvement leads to anticipation, and vice versa. A spirit of sociable competition can be exploited and carried over from the creation of funny hats from scraps, or the exchange of knitting or leather-work patterns, to the achievement of greater independence. Residents will endure considerable physical effort for social compensations. In this regard, the July 1962 issue of the

Bulletin of the Institute of Gerontology carried a supplemental article titled "A Rewarding Year's Experience in a Recreation Program" by Mrs. Fannie Rector,[4] who writes to this point. This article describes the activities program which she established at Rest View Convalescent Home in Des Moines, Iowa. Such a program requires the expenditure of greater amounts of interest and concern for people than of money.

When I decided to include Process and Procedure in my list of "P's," I separated them in order to distinguish the disease process from the rehabilitative procedure. Each of these areas is vast enough to occupy practitioners of the medical and physical therapies for a lifetime, so I do not propose to treat them in any depth here. However, it is useful to know as much as one can about the processes with which one must deal. Recognizing that certain diagnoses apparently carry with them certain behaviors seems to make them more tolerable to the worker and to the family, although let me say that they need not be accepted as inevitable and permanent. It will also increase the positive factors in workers' motivation to know what can reasonably be expected and how long they must persist in order to achieve the desired goals. The differences in the kinds of arthritis provides an example here. X-rays of the joint, in both rheumatoid and degenerative arthritis (osteoarthritis), show narrowed joint space, but the appearance presented by the rheumatic joint is reddened shiny skin, covering a swollen painful joint, of which the patient will be very protective. The osteoarthritic joint, on the other hand, will not be red or shiny, nor so obviously swollen and will not elicit the same protective mechanisms in the patient. In both cases heat and exercise are used (these and all other treatments are, of course, supervised by the physician), but with the rheumatoid arthritic splints may be applied to prevent deformity, or progression in deformity.

To know the tremendous psychological impact that severe cardiac and circulatory dysfunction has upon a person increases the ability to work with this person. The significance of the heart, and the brain—the centers of life and control—can hardly be exaggerated, and, of course, the anxiety which accompanies the threat to either is very great. It is not surprising, then, that frequently the hemiplegic patient is preoccupied with himself and his illness; that he is constantly tense, clings to others for help; that he misinterprets the reality of his illness and the extent to which he can exert himself or should avoid any form of exertion; that he allows others to make all decisions for him, and so on. These reactions make him a more difficult person to rehabilitate than the patient with a fractured hip, for example, and greater persistence in motivation will be required. However, the job can be done with less frustration when such knowledge is available.

Aphasia, so often a concomitant of hemiplegia, presents its own exquisite frustrations for the patient, for his family, and for those who work with him. Since language is the commonest means of communication and therefore of maintaining social networks, its loss is a grievous blow. The frustration of knowing, but being unable to express what one wishes to convey, or of being unable to recognize meaning in the words addressed to one, is very threatening and very severe. Unfortunately, the common tendency is to treat those who cannot speak as if they could not hear either, or perhaps as if they had suddenly lost all intelligence, when it is a matter of having lost ability to express the product of the intelligence. Rather than shouting at, or isolating these patients, the worker and the patient's family can develop a simple form of communication. If the patient has expressive aphasia—that is, if he can understand but cannot speak—the worker can reduce the patient's tension by asking questions structured in such a way that the patient can nod "yes" and "no," or perhaps he can manage these two words only. Signs also can be developed and used for frequent requests such as a bedpan, or a drink, or to be moved. To keep the patient involved with life outside himself, the worker can talk casually and calmly, clearly and deliberately, about current interests and activities in the home rather than about the past or future. One of the characteristics of hemiplegia is lability (instability) and contemplation of the future which at the moment seems so bleak, frequently produces tears, which further distress the patient and, usually, the worker.

If the patient does not recognize the meaning of words spoken to him (receptive aphasia) one helpful tool is a series of cards with useful pictures drawn or pasted on them. The patient can recognize the items pictured when he is unable to recognize the word symbols for them. If the word is printed below the picture, the patient may be able to relearn the connection similarly to the way a child learns words. Repetition of words in connection with items is also useful and need not take extra time. Nouns are the earliest words to return and probably the most useful; next are verbs; and the last words are the prepositions and little connecting words which are usually the least important in making one's needs and concerns known. The patient who is unable to converse easily is quickly isolated, unless specific effort is made to avoid this development.

PROCEDURES

Procedures (the last of six P's), and techniques, vary greatly from one institution to another. Each physician has certain patterns of treatment he has found effective. Since one of the nurse's functions is to complete the medical restoration, the nursing activities will, of course, be based upon the physician's plan of care. The two greatest concerns in developing independent self-care in residents are feeding and controlled elimination. The book *Nursing Home Management* by Williams *et al.*[5] illustrates many useful contrivances to help the disabled person. It is even better if the patient, especially the hemiplegic, can be taught early to feed himself without these aids. This and toothbrushing, hair brushing and combing, helping with the bed bath, etc, should start as soon as the patient emerges from the acutely ill phase. Prior to this, the nurse can do passive range-of-motion exercises and position the patient to keep joints functional. These patients, and the arthritics, require great persistence and a recognition on a realistic level of their potential. No one can delineate absolute goals for the patient; his potential and response to treatment are often unpredictable and are the governing factors in the rehabilitation program.

In establishing control of elimination a program should be set up within twenty-four to thirty-six hours of a cerebral vascular accident. There is no physiological reason for incontinence in most hemiplegic patients, unlike those with traumatic paraplegia. I have already identified some of the contributory emotional factors. A regular schedule of elimination is among the first steps; exercise is another. Patients often can be trained to defecate by using a commode when they cannot seem to manage to do so with a bedpan. The usual sitting position assumed on a commode also contributes to better performance. Diet, including adequate fluid intake (i.e., 2,000 cc), fruits, roughage, and so on also contributes. Preventing distention of the bladder or of the bowel by impaction will reduce atony (weakness) of the muscles involved in elimination. The patient's desire to remain dry is essential for successful control. If the workers do not accept incontinence as an inevitability, but institute a plan for control at once, the patient's motivation will be reinforced. You know how embarrassed the patient is with the first such accident. Let us capitalize on this attitude. Other accidents of a similar nature will happen but their frequency can be gradually reduced. Also use knowledge gleaned about the patient's past habits. A schedule based on these will be more likely to succeed. Awareness of the environment seems to increase as patients begin wearing street clothes. Whether they adopt a more independent role when thus dressed than when in a hospital shirt, I don't know. I suspect that they do, but perhaps this only coincides with increased exercise and muscle strength. I do know that whatever training plan is made for controlling elimination, it requires that the patient participate, that the workers use a consistent (not stereotyped) approach, and that everyone involved believes the end justifies the time expenditure. Moreover, I believe that there are few physicians who do not welcome requests for permission to institute restorative measures for the benefit of their patients, or who are not willing to take time, if necessary, to demonstrate the physical measures they wish to have carried out.

The social activities programs lie within the area of the nurse's supplemental functions, but they have therapeutic effects which contribute to whatever restorative program the physician will approve. There are many resources available to those who wish to inform themselves about rehabilitative measures which do not require the specialized preparation of the physical therapist. The Department of Health, Education, and Welfare of the United States Government has developed two booklets which are available from the Government Printing Office, Washington 25, D.C. (*Strike Back at Stroke* and *Strike Back at Arthritis.*) The New York State Department of Health, Albany, New York, publishes a booklet titled *Management of the Patient with Hemiplegia,* which is directed to those responsible for the care of hemiplegic patients. These booklets are profusely illustrated with range-of-motion exercises suitable for preventing deformities related to the conditions. Some have more written content than others. And, of course, the volume *Nursing Home Management* will be found very helpful. As a rule, state departments of health have on their staffs consultants in physical therapy, nursing, nutrition, and mental health, whose work it is, at least in part, to respond to requests for assistance from nursing home administrators.

If you are thinking of establishing a more active rehabilitation plan than has been in use heretofore, remember that for the staff as well as for the patients, it will require learning and changed behavior. Greatest resistance to change is in the area of nursing, where much must be unlearned before new philosophy and approaches can be accepted and acted upon. An ongoing in-service program increases the interest, knowledge, and capabilities of staff more effectively than an all-out big effort. Large expenditures of money are not essential, neither are additions to the staff of an occupational or physical therapist. Mrs. Rector's article (mentioned earlier) demonstrates what can be done with a little guidance and a lot of concern for the people who are patients or residents, guests, or clients. Definite techniques to be used, rather than the generalized concepts I have mentioned, are most acceptable to workers. These techniques, with specific variations, can then be used with patients designated by the physician. It is wise to start with a few potentially highly responsive patients, so that workers and patients enjoy success.

The essential thing in caring for definitely disabled patients is to help them regain the use of their utmost capabilities. With regard to the restorative process, the therapist must believe absolutely and enthusiastically that, in the long run, rehabilitation pays the biggest dividends, in both the tangibles and intangibles. Attitudes are caught, not taught. Above all, they are caught from the administrator and the nursing personnel in the home. A good example of this is to be found in the story of Rancho Los Amigos, the hospital whose Attending Staff Association produced the important book *Nursing Home*

Administration.[6] The Rancho started out as the county poor farm. The beginnings of its transformation are told in an article in the June 1958 issue of *Nursing Outlook,* "Rehabilitating Patients with Chronic Disease." It is a dramatic account of the determination of two women to overcome the residents' lethargy and apathetic acceptance of their status, and the lack of understanding of potentials on the part of the staff. Because they believed strongly that each man has the right and the duty to function to the limit of his capacity, an amazing number of their patients did just that. A similar course of staff-patient involvement will, I believe, always pay big dividends.

FOOTNOTES

1. Zane, M. D. and Lowenthal M., "Motivation in Rehabilitation of the Physically Handicapped," *Archives of Physical Medicine and Rehabilitation,* 41:9:400–7, September 1960.
2. Landau, Gertrude, "Restoration of Self-Esteem," *Geriatrics,* 10:3:141–43, March 1955.
3. Kelman, Howard R., "An Experiment in Rehabilitation of Nursing Home Patients," *Public Health Reports,* 77:4:356–66, April 1962.
4. Rector, Fannie, "A Rewarding Year's Experience in a Recreation Program," Supplement – *Bulletin of the Institute of Gerontology, Adding Life to Years,* University of Iowa, 9:7:3–6, July 1962.
5. Williams, R. C. *et al., Nursing Home Management.* New York: McGraw-Hill, 1959.
6. Gerletti, John D. *et al. Nursing Home Administration.* Downey, California: Attending Staff Association, 1961.

ADDITIONAL READINGS

7. Buchwald, Edith, *Physical Rehabilitation for Daily Living,* New York: McGraw-Hill, 1952.
8. Hackley, John A., "Instructing Nursing Home Personnel in Rehabilitation Techniques," *Public Health Reports,* 74:2:989–94, November 1959.
9. Miller, Clara H. and Hamil, Evelyn M., "Rehabilitating Patients with Chronic Disease." *Nursing Outlook,* 58:6:324–25, June 1958.
10. Shoutz, F. C. and Fink, S. L. "A Method for Evaluating Psychological Adjustment of the Chronically Ill." *American Journal of Physical Medicine,* 40:2:63–69, April 1961.
11. Wohl, Michael G. (ed.), *Long Term Illness: Management of the Chronically Ill Patient.* Philadelphia: W. B. Saunders, 1959.

Part Three

REHABILITATION

Chapter 7

Procedures in Rehabilitation

WILLIAM D. PAUL, *M.D.* and TERRY B. JONES, *R.P.T.*

The nonambulatory individual poses problems common to all of us whether we work in clinics, nursing homes, or hospitals—small or large. The important thing to consider is that most of these people can overcome at least some of their functional loss. Early exercises can often be started in bed. Some of the simplest activities such as moving from one side of the bed to the other and rolling over are actually important in the strengthening of the arms and body. To be able to sit up in bed also is an essential achievement leading to ambulation. The strength and balance which are developed by these activities make it possible for the patient to increase his or her independence in their activities of daily living much sooner.

The loss of use of one or more extremities often makes it necessary for the individual to have help in making transfers from the bed to a chair or from chair to toilet or into a bathtub.

Some people can improve so that they can begin ambulation with assistance and may be carefully fitted with crutches for added stabilization. Owing to the many body types which must be fitted, however, each individual must be carefully measured and the crutches tried out to make sure that the patient actually walks with the best possible gait considering the disability.

MEASURING FOR CRUTCHES

In measuring a patient for crutches, the height of the crutches and the level of the hand piece are primary considerations. If the crutches are too long, they force the shoulders up and the patient has no way of pushing his body off the floor, but, more importantly, the crutch that is too long may cause injury to the nerves under the armpit. If the crutches are too short, the patient leans forward too far and stands poorly.

Many methods are used for measuring the patient for crutches. Three procedures with the patient lying supine in bed are suggested here:

1. The crutch length is measured from the anterior fold of the axilla to a point 6 inches (15 cm.) out from the lateral side of the heel.
2. The crutch length is measured from the anterior fold of the axilla to the lateral side of the heel, and 2 inches (5 cm.) are added.
3. If the patient wears braces and crutches, the crutch tips and tops are placed on the crutches and the crutch length is then measured from the anterior fold of the axilla and about two to three fingers below the apex of the axilla to the lateral side of the heel of the shoe.

Fitting the crutches in the supine position is only a working basis to gauge the approximate crutch length. In order to make the final adjustments for correct crutch length, the patient must be in the standing position.

The person to be measured for crutches should be standing. The top of the crutch should be 1 inch below the axilla (with the shoulders relaxed) and the tip of the crutch approximately 6 inches out to the side and forward of each foot. An extremely tall adult would need the crutches out to the side and forward of each foot perhaps as much as 14 or 15 inches, whereas a short adult or small child would require a smaller base of support and should be fitted with the crutch tips 6 inches or less to the side and forward of each foot. The hand piece should be positioned at a height which positions the elbows with a bend of 30 degrees.

IN AND OUT OF BATHTUB

Preliminary exercises: from bed to wheelchair; from wheelchair to chair, to toilet, to mat.

Into bathtub:

Starting position: Patient should sit in wheelchair, approach bathtub from side near free end of tub. Lock brakes. Be sure to leave enough space between wheelchair and tub so that legs can be lifted without bruising them.

Instructions (directed to the patient):

1. Lift left leg with both hands over edge of tub.
2. Lift right leg with both hands over edge of tub and . . .
3. . . . place it next to left leg.
4. Unlock brakes. Place wheelchair as close as possible to tub, so that your legs hang over the edge of tub. Lock brakes and slide as far forward on wheelchair seat as possible.
5. Place right hand on far edge of tub and left hand on left armrest.
6. Shift right hand to opposite edge of tub, while therapist grasps you around waist. Keep left hand on left armrest or place it . . .

7. . . . on edge of tub next to you. Push hard on both hands and lower body slowly into tub. *Slow* bending of elbows will control movement.

Out of bathtub: Reverse entire procedure.

Precautions: To prevent sliding, a rubber mat with suction cups should be placed on bottom of tub. While patient lowers his body into tub it is important (a) to support him around waist (b) to avoid a sudden stretch in shoulder joint by bending elbows as slowly as possible (c) to guide patient's legs if he is very tall, and also if he is spastic. (The same precautions have to be taken when getting out of tub.) If there are sensory disturbances, extreme caution has to be observed as to water temperature.

Helpful remarks: A small stool can be placed in tub, so there is less height to be overcome when getting in and out of tub. To prevent slipping, suction crutch tips should be placed on legs of stool and stool should stand on a rubber mat which also has suction cups. If tub is filled with water, it is easier to get in and out, but great caution must be observed.

It is essential to place wheelchair as close to tub as possible, to facilitate getting in and out of tub. Placement of wheelchair will depend on the layout of bathroom and kind of tub used.

If the tub is flush against the wall, it will be helpful to attach a horizontal bar to wall, so that patient can grasp it and push on it when getting in and out. If wheelchair cannot be brought near enough to tub and/or if armrests are not removable, a small bench will bridge gap between wheelchair and tub.

FROM WHEELCHAIR DIRECTLY TO TOILET SEAT AND BACK

The transfer from wheelchair to toilet seat is basically the same as transfer from wheelchair to chair. The following method is most commonly used. Placement of wheelchair will vary with layout of different bathrooms (see variations below).

Preliminary exercises: sitting balanced; push-ups; from wheelchair to chair.

From wheelchair to toilet seat:

Starting position: Patient should sit in wheelchair. Roll as close as possible to toilet seat, approaching same from the side. Footrests are down. (May also be up—will depend on shape of toilet bowl.)

Instructions (directed to the patient):

1. Place both legs with hands toward right of wheelchair. Slide to edge of chair, grasping both armrests.
2. Place left hand on toilet seat (or pipe or toilet tank), still grasping right armrest with right hand. Push on both hands . . .
3. . . . and lift and shift body onto toilet seat, turning at the same time until . . .

4. . . . you are straight.

From toilet seat to wheelchair: Reverse entire procedure.

Precautions: If lower extremities are very spastic, therapist guides them to prevent bruising of toes and feet.

For additional support and to ensure balance when sliding onto toilet seat and back or when sitting on it, the following can be done:

a. Patient holds onto wheelchair and/or iron bar alongside wall.
b. A chair is placed in front of patient with backrest facing him so that back can be grasped for support.
c. Wheelchair is placed in front of patient with armrestsf acing him so that armrests can be grasped. Many patients find this position helpful when using toilet paper.
d. If toilet has a tank it can be used as a backrest.

If patient tends to have pressure sores, a foam-rubber ring should be placed on toilet seat.

Helpful remarks: Most patients find it easier to adjust their clothes while sitting in wheelchair before and after using toilet.

Variations in placement of wheelchair:

a. Wheelchair is placed alongside toilet, if armrests are removable, so that patient slides or lifts himself sideways onto toilet.
b. Wheelchair is rolled as close as possible facing toilet so that patient slides forward onto same, in a straddling position and backward into wheelchair.
c. Wheelchair is backed up to toilet if there is a zipper in backrest.

FROM BED TO WHEELCHAIR AND BACK—
Wheelchair at angle (nonremovable armrests)

This method is the most common one. It can be used by patients with or without braces.

Preliminary exercises: sitting up; sitting balanced; moving forward and backward while sitting; push-ups; and sitting with legs over edge of bed.

Equipment: bed, wheelchair.

From bed to wheelchair:

Starting position: Wheelchair is placed at slight angle along right side of bed and facing forward. Footrests are down and brakes locked.

Instructions (directed to the patient):

1. Sit with legs over edge of bed. Place left hand behind left hip on bed and right hand on right armrest. Turn body slightly to right.
2. Push on both hands, raise body and lift yourself across and down . . .
3. . . . into chair. Place feet on footrests.

From wheelchair to bed: Reverse entire procedure.

Instructions (directed to the patient):

1. Sit in wheelchair along right side of bed facing forward and at a slight angle.
2. Place right hand on armrest and left hand on bed near left hip. Push on both hands, raise body, and lift yourself across . . .
3. . . . and onto bed. Slide back on bed as far as necessary. Lift legs up with hands.

FROM BED TO WHEELCHAIR AND BACK—
Wheelchair alongside bed (removable armrests)

From bed to wheelchair:

Starting position: Remove armrest, and place chair alongside and as close as possible to bed. Lock brakes.

Instructions (directed to the patient):

Place right hand next to right hip on bed and left hand on left armrest. Push on both hands, slide (or lift) sideways onto chair. Attach armrest. Place feet on footrests.

From wheelchair to bed: Reverse entire procedure.

Starting position: Sit in wheelchair along side of bed as close as possible.

Instructions (directed to the patient):

Remove right armrest, place it on bed. Place right hand near right hip on bed and grasp left armrest with left hand. Push on both hands and slide (or lift yourself) onto bed.

Precautions: To prevent tipping no weight should be on footrests. If possible, both feet, or at least one foot, should be on floor. There is more weight on the arm that is on the bed. In the beginning, the therapist stands by ready to give support around waist.

Helpful remarks: When getting from wheelchair to bed, the chair should be moved to the right distance from headboard, so that when the patient slides into bed he can lie down without having to move up or down in bed. This is especially true for very heavy patients.

Instead of placing armrest on bed, it may also be hung on handle of back of wheelchair.

This outline suggests activities in which it is most important that the patient develop some degree of independence. We can see, too, that each activity is in itself good exercise if the patient is encouraged to carry it through himself. By progressively demanding more of an individual, we encourage him to help himself and ultimately we all gain by his increased functional ability.

Chapter 8

Clothing: Social and Therapeutic Values

ADELINE M. HOFFMAN, *Ph.D.*

The domain of clothing and fashion has been invaded by experts in every field of study from art to international trade, including business, home economics, psychology, economics, anthropology, literature, and the theater. Clothing is of great importance to people, as a means of social identification and as a source of personal satisfaction. George Hartman, professor of psychology at Columbia University, called clothing a "persistent center of interest in everyone's life." Though it varies greatly in intensity and expression, Hartman contends that it is a fundamental life interest. Yet most people make an "essentially superficial approach to this ever recurring topic, as though a feeling of being engaged in the trivial were inseparable from it." Clothing has always been regarded as one of the three essential needs of people, the other two being food and shelter, but it has been only recently that clothing has been given much consideration by the social scientists, or that we have recognized the "social science" aspects of clothing.

Social scientists, however, are coming to see that there are positive psychological values in being well dressed at any age and in any environment. The desire for approval is present in people of all ages—children, adolescents, adults, and older people. Thus it is often said that we dress for other people—for their approval—and that in this approval we find our sense of well-being and self-confidence, as well as our feeling of social acceptance.

In his book, *The Importance of Wearing Clothes,* Lawrence Langner writes that "one of the greatest spiritual needs of people is the admiration of their fellow men and women and here clothing plays a major role." Even Thorstein Veblen, in his famous classic of economic thought, *The Theory of the Leisure Class,* wrote that "the need for dress is eminently a 'higher' or spiritual need," and pointed out the relationship of dress to canons of good taste and reputability. And Ralph Waldo Emerson, noted American writer, in his essay on "Social Aims," had a word to say about clothing. After discussing manners, he said, "I have heard with admiring submission the experience of the lady who declared that 'the sense of being well dressed gives a feeling of inward tranquility which religion is powerless to bestow.' "

These expressions of the significance of clothing are illustrated over and over in the experience of people. An older woman who had to be hospitalized for a time was made to wear the typical white hospital gown and she said she did not want any visitors while she had to wear such a garment. When she was allowed to put on a pretty nightgown and negligee or bed jacket, she removed the ban on visitors. Thus she was expressing what clothing meant to her. Another woman exhibited the same sort of sensitivity in a different way. She had just come to live in a retirement home. Shortly thereafter, she got in touch with her grandson and told him that she would have to have more and better clothing if she were to associate comfortably with the other women in the home.

What is there about clothing, then, that makes it so important to people, and why do people feel differently when they are dressed well? Why do men want to dress their wives as expensively as they can? Why do women ask what other women are going to wear, when a special social event is announced? And why do we wear certain clothing for special occasions? The answer to these questions is that we do these things as an expression of our efforts to observe custom and tradition in regard to the use of clothing. Moreover, if we go back into literature, we find that clothing has always been, as it is today, a kind of status symbol. Shakespeare makes numerous references to clothing, the most familiar of which is the one from Hamlet in which he says, "Costly thy habit as thy purse can buy; but not expressed in fancy; rich, not gaudy; for apparel oft proclaims the man." And Veblen, again, in his chapter, "Dress as an Expression of the Pecuniary Culture," says, "Probably at no other point is the sense of shabbiness so keenly felt as it is if we fall short of the standards set by social usage in this matter of dress."

CLOTHING PROMOTES THE PERSON

Perhaps more important to the individual than his "feeling" about clothing is that it can become an expression of his personality; an extention of himself. In his frequently quoted work on the psychology of clothes, George Dearborn refers to the relationship between clothing and personality thus, 'We might consider clothes as a vicarious artificial skin, almost an extension of the individual boundary, involving important relationships between the person and his environment, spiritual as much as material."

Clothing, then, is an expression of the aesthetic sensitivity of the wearer and it serves also as a morale builder. It has often been said that when a woman is a bit discouraged or low in spirits, it is time for her to go out and buy a new hat. Perhaps there is some wisdom in this aphorism for we know the morale-building value of new clothes. There are some women who buy clothes just for the vicarious pleasure the buying itself gives them. A few days later they return the garments to the stores.

One of the things most women, as well as children, love about clothes is the possibility that other people will like their selections and express their approval, through well-worded compliments. This kind of morale building, through compliments on clothing, lends itself very well to nursing and retirement home situations, but care must be taken in the wording of such expressions of approval, lest they sound like sheer judgments rather than compliments. Consider, for a moment, the person who said, "that's the best-looking dress I have ever seen you wear," as if to express disapproval of all the other dresses in the person's wardrobe. Another might say, "I always liked that coat," as if to imply that it is really time to get a new one. To compliment one person in a group of three is, of course, to slight the other two, particularly if you compliment one or her pretty new hair style and you ignore the pretty new hair styles of the other two people.

It is always a greater compliment to talk about how attractive the person looks wearing the pretty garment, rather than talking about the garment itself. The wearer might think the compliment should be accorded the family member from whom the garment was received as a gift, rather than for herself. Compliments must be used sparingly and with evident sincerity to carry the most weight. Thus compliments given too freely may ring of their insincerity, such as terms of endearment used generally as personal pronouns.

GOOD APPEARANCE RAISES MORALE

Since attractive clothing is important, not only to the wearer but also to the observer, let us consider what we really mean by attractive clothing. The elements of attractiveness are color, style, fabric, decorativeness, and distinctiveness, all of which contribute to setting each individual apart from others. Attractiveness in clothing, even in a nursing home or retirement home environment, carries with it a kind of aesthetic stimulation, just as does a beautiful sunset, a beautiful flower, or a beautiful person. Philosophers of art tell us that the function of beauty is to "lift the human spirit." Many people in nursing and retirement homes could do with having their spirits lifted a bit and clothing can well serve this function.

To get the most out of clothing in this way, people must be sensitive to their surroundings, for clothing is the immediate environment of the individual; and it becomes also a part of the total situation for all other people. Sprucing up awakens one's spirits. When a woman knows she is looking her best, she feels like a more important and worthwhile person. Not only does good appearance do this for the individual but it commands the respect of others, and gives one a feeling of a continuing grasp on life. This is forcefully illustrated in the case of the woman who dressed up to preside at her club luncheon, though she was known to be gravely ill at the time.

The tone of a social occasion is often set by the clothes people wear, and thus a commonplace social function can take on greater importance for the guests in accordance with the "dressing up." In a nursing home or retirement home situation, a bit of "fixing up," or even a change of clothing, can make a social event out of coming together for afternoon tea or other mid-meal refreshment. In a nursing home where one of the patients was expecting a visit from her grandson she was decked out with a ribbon in her hair and this little touch of decoration made her feel dressed up, and, as she said, "made the day for her." And speaking of decoration, the greatest compliment for an individual is a flower—a single flower; not a flower put in a container of water on the bedside table, but a flower pinned on the dress, or even the bed jacket of the patient, just as we pin an orchid on the wife of the speaker in the receiving line, or at the banquet table. Flowers speak a language all their own which everyone understands. I am reminded of the pushcart peddler in New York who had a sign on his pushcart that said, "Wear a flower this morning and you'll feel important all day." He sold his flowers long before the other flower peddlers. You know how you feel when you go to a restaurant or hotel dining room where there are flowers on all the tables but the one where you are seated. You feel a bit cheated or left out. In Europe, flowers are used much more than in the United States to express courtesies and to decorate home and persons. We should use them more.

There is very little eventfulness in the lives of most patients in nursing homes and even in some retirement homes, but the little there is can be highlighted by a bit of dressing up in anticipation of events, even such simple ones as entertainment provided by community singing groups. Through such dressing up the individual contributes to the environment and experiences a sense of personal participation in the event. To add to the enjoyment of holidays in nursing homes and retirement homes a little dressing up is always in order. To help mark the special holidays a few touches can be added, such as a tiny green-and-white shamrock for St. Patrick's day pinned on the dress, bed jacket, or robe of the individual patient, the small Christmas decoration at Christmas, even though there is a decorated Christmas tree in sight, and for the Fourth of July, a little bow of red, white, and blue ribbon, like a sorority pledge ribbon. This touch of decoration for the individual patient can provide a sense of participation in the celebration that goes on in the outside world and create an air of festivity.

Color is an important element in the attractiveness of clothing. Just as fashion in clothing changes, so does fashion in color. There was a time when it was considered proper and in good taste for older ladies to wear black, gray, or dark, subdued shades of other colors. For women well past the bloom of youth, these dark colors emphasize their own lack of color in their complexions and in their hair. Colors more appropriate for older women, in terms of enhancing whatever personal coloring they have, are the pastels. Not only are they more cheerful and easier to look at; they are kinder to the skin and hair tones of older women. They suggest sunshine, laughter, and lightheartedness, rather than the somber gloom created by the darker shades. The same is true of decorating colors used in the nursing home environment. Color affects mood; thus change in a color worn can change a mood. Variety of color in the clothing of the geriatric patient can be very beneficial.

Under favorable conditions, daytime clothing should be worn in preference to bedtime clothing or lounging clothing, to create a feeling of recovery to normal health rather than that of being sick. People in nursing and retirement homes should have some opportunity to choose their own clothing, since choice in itself has the therapeutic values of achievement and personal control. In some nursing home situations, almost every move a patient makes and almost all that is done for him becomes a matter of routine in which he has little or no choice and no opportunity for expression of individuality and taste.

LINK WITH THE OUTSIDE WORLD THROUGH NEW CLOTHING

Everyone loves new clothes and even though nursing home patients may have little opportunity, if any, to go out, there is something about new clothes that is important to such people. New clothes create a feeling of anticipation; of looking ahead into the future, rather than backward to the past, when old clothing was new and in style. The latest style, provided it is appropriate, gives a woman a feeling of being up-to-date. This in itself is one of the most important therapeutic values of clothing; it is a link with the outside world and a sense of the future, rather than the past.

Patients in nursing homes, of course, have less need for new clothes than people in good health in normal social life. However, for all people, there are certain values in newness. Some old people cling to their old clothes because there is little opportunity to obtain new ones, or because old things are familiar and provide a sense of relationship to their environment, while newness may be suspect. Still other old people experience a childish sense of excitement over anything that is new. It is likely that patients who are mentally alert will find greater interest and satisfaction in the element of newness than will others who may be apathetic and thus fail to find much stimulation in new clothes.

GROOMING THERAPY

Did you ever observe how women feel when they have just had their hair done at a beauty salon? This beauty treatment gives them, at least momentarily, a sort of new lease on life. Good grooming, cleanliness, and care of the hair would do as much for women in nursing and retirement homes. Some provision should be made for grooming therapy, either by having facilities and personnel in the home, or through special arrangement with a local beauty shop or other resources appropriate to the needs of the patients in a nursing home or guests in a retirement home. Minimum care for women not able to take care of their own needs would be daily combing and arranging of the hair and shampooing as needed. When people see each other well groomed, they all benefit in a therapeutic sense.

PRACTICAL CONSIDERATIONS

In addition to the social and therapeutic values of clothing, there are a few practical aspects that should be considered. One of the most important of these is comfort. No clothing fits correctly nor is it a good choice, if it is uncomfortable or difficult to get into. There are women who have physical handicaps of varying degrees who cannot use conventional clothing. However, for these women there is clothing designed to meet their special needs and catalogues of such clothing are available. One source is the Rehabilitation Center for Vocational and Rehabilitation Services, 2239 East Fifty-fifth Street, Cleveland, Ohio. The garments and other related items available from this source are functional, attractive, and moderate in cost.

Another important consideration in the care of clothing is adequate laundering and attention to such details as replacing missing buttons, and making such minor repairs as may be needed for maximum use of clothing. To facilitate sorting after laundering, all clothing should be clearly marked with the name of the owner. Since laundering is done by machine rather than by hand, all clothing should be machine washable and should not require any special care in laundering. Friends and relatives who may be greatly devoted to the persons in nursing and retirement homes may be very impractical in their choice of clothing items as gifts. Sometimes the clothing items they select are so fancy that they seem out-of-place and consequently are never worn. This is especially true of fancy lingerie. Rather than making their selections on the basis of their own taste and the clothing they would like for themselves, they need to take into consideration the special needs and tastes of the older women. The element of appropriateness is, of course, also true of clothing for older men, though there are fewer problems with men's clothing.

Fashion of the last quarter of a century reveals changes not only in fashion in clothing but also in standards of modesty. Many of the women in nursing homes today were born in the 1880's and 1890's. They grew up before such feminine fashion innovations as the strapless evening dress, short shorts for daytime wear and the bikini bathing suit. The standards of modesty that these women lived with became part of their personal standards, and many of them cannot accept today's standards, although other women do accept them and are not disturbed by them. Those who do hold to rigid standards of modesty should be accorded the dignity of making their own choices and should be provided with appropriate bed attire and a robe of some kind for time spent out of bed. What may be taken in stride by one older woman of today may be regarded as embarrassing exposure by an older woman who has maintained the strict standards of her earlier years. It must never be forgotten that pride, dignity, and one's personal standards are still important as a means of expressing a sense of personal worth of the individual.

PERSONAL APPEARANCE AS A CLUE TO MENTAL HEALTH

The therapeutic value of clothing was dramatically demonstrated by the Fashion Group of San Francisco, working in cooperation with the San Francisco Association of Mental Health in a fashion therapy project for women patients at the Napa State Hospital. The Fashion Group is a professional organization of women in the field of retail clothing merchandising, and allied fields, with units in twenty-five cities in the United States and five countries. The fashion therapy was an effort to prepare mental patients about to be discharged to return to normal community life, by bringing them up-to-date in fashion and helping them to improve their personal appearance. The therapy included attractive hair styling, effective use of cosmetics, and advantageous use of clothing. The project was so successful at the California hospital that the superintendent decided the therapy should be made available to women who had not responded to any treatment, in addition to those about to be released. Since 1959, when the project was started in San Francisco, it has spread to eleven cities in the United States, and Paris. It has long been observed generally that mental patients who show some signs of caring about their appearance are beginning to get a grip on themselves and are on the road to recovery. The Fashion Group project, however, was the first organized effort in this area of therapy. One of the results of the project at the California hospital was that men patients started to spruce up, nurses improved their appearance, and there was a marked increase in beauty salon patronage at the hospital. Also, full-length mirrors were installed in the wards. Though clothing is generally regarded as a status symbol, it is more than that; it is an expression of the self-image and a continual means of self-renewal.

REFERENCES

1. Dearborn, George Van Ness, "The Psychology of Clothing." *Psychological Monograph*, 26:1: 1–72, 1918–19.
2. Hartman, George W., "Clothing: Personal Problem and Social Issue." *Journal of Home Economics,* 41:6: 295–98, June 1949.
3. Langner, Lawrence, *The Importance of Wearing Clothes.* New York: Hastings House, 1959.
4. Thomson, Thelma, "Fashion Therapy." *Journal of Home Economics,* 54:10: 835–36, December 1962.
5. Veblen, Thorstein, *The Theory of the Leisure Class.* New York: New American Library (Mentor), 1954.

Part Four

NUTRITION AND FOOD SERVICE

Chapter 9

Diets for the Elderly

MARGARET A. OHLSON, *Ph.D.*

METHUSELAH

Methuselah ate what he found on his plate,
And never, as people do now,
Did he note the amount of the calory count;
He ate it because it was chow.
He wasn't disturbed as at dinner he sat,
Devouring a roast or a pie,
To think it was lacking in granular fat
Or a couple of vitamins shy.
He cheerfully chewed each species of food,
Unmindful of troubles or fears
Lest his health might be hurt
By some fancy dessert;
And he lived over nine hundred years.

— UNKNOWN

It would be interesting to know what Methuselah ate, but it would be equally interesting to know what he was like during his life span.

One of the real problems in evaluating the food needed by older persons is the lack of a standard of what constitutes a well-nourished adult. With the increase in variability among people as they grow older, this lack of standard is even more important. The midwestern farmer, feeding cattle for market, has a clear-cut picture of a well-finished market animal and his feeding plans are structured to create this animal. In feeding man, we obviously are interested in longevity rather than market finish, and the required diet undoubtedly is quite different. We know from animal experiments that if we start in childhood, underfeeding will increase the life span but unfortunately most of the increased time accrues before puberty. For man, longevity without the ability to compete in an adult world could be burdensome.

We express differences in adults by such generalized terms as "well nourished," vigorous, flabby, lacking in vitality, and tend to be baffled by the patient who is chronically tired but has no evidence of disease to explain the symptoms. Many social and emotional factors may have contributed to the general lack of health of this patient but the probabilities are that decreased motivation has resulted in reduced intake of food, even though the patient may be ingesting enough calories to support unwanted pounds of weight. A prescription for vitamins seldom solves the problem.

In this country, there is little frank deficiency disease but many older people reach a stage where chronic undernutrition is expressed as a general lack of well-being. A few examples will illustrate the point. Some years ago, a woman was referred to us for instruction in a diet to bring about a twenty-five–pound weight loss. She was a flabby, white, unthrifty-looking woman with obvious lack of energy but she was not obviously edematous. She had been treated for more than a year for a persistent normocytic anemia with all of the usual iron and vitamin combinations including injections. There had been some temporary improvement but no prolonged remission. Her diet history suggested erratic eating with emphasis on sugars and sweets but little good-quality protein. She was given a diet generous in protein, largely from animal sources, but with a moderate number of calories. She complained bitterly that we were forcing her to eat so much that she would not lose weight. The first six weeks on the diet justified her interpretation as no weight was lost, although her appearance improved and she obviously felt better. At this time, she started to excrete an increased amount of urine. During three days she lost fifteen pounds. She also lost much of her appearance of flabbiness and both the red cell count and the hemoglobin increased to within normal values. For the next few weeks she continued to lose slowly and was eventually stabilized on an intake of food suitable for her age and activity with emphasis on good-quality protein.

One of the few things about which scientists agree in feeding older people is that the weight should be within normal limits. A year later this woman had required no further treatment for the anemia, was well and active, and had maintained her weight. We have recently had a similar experience with a 60-year-old man who was admitted with a mild case of decompensation of the heart. He lost thirty pounds in about two weeks and yet he did not have obvious edema when admitted.

Weight loss is always difficult to achieve but it may be particularly discouraging in the older person whose weight may be the result of years of poor eating practices. There is little doubt that the patients described were building lean tissue at the same time that fat was being burned. The prompt remission of the anemia in the woman is a key to this concept as is the fact that this type of response to high-protein, calorie-restricted diet in a flabby adult is always associated with a reduction in dress size and an appearance of improved muscle tone before weight losses can be measured by the scales. It is easy for both the doctor and the patient to become discouraged before these adjustments are complete and to give up rather than persist in the diet. Diets of 1,000 calories per day for an average-sized adult may provide calorie-to-protein ratios too low for retention of protein to occur and replacement of lean tissue may therefore not take place in the flabby patient. Weight is lost with difficulty and without improvement in well-being. A more generous intake of calories will mean slower weight losses but a patient with poor muscle tone and limited vitality who loses weight on a balanced diet always has an increased sense of well-being after several weeks of dieting.

The type of diet used is essentially one of normal foods with the omission only of sweet desserts and the extra fat which occurs in fried food or fat which is added as seasoning, such as sour cream, whipped cream, heavy mayonnaise, and the like. A pat of table spread is given each meal for the bread and for seasoning vegetables. Food is served in three to five meals of about equal size.

While it is generally accepted that total calories must be reduced with increasing age and reduced activity if undesirable weight gains are to be avoided, it is not as well understood that nutrients and calories occur together in foods and a perscription eat less is apt to be interpreted as less of everything. The diet described can form the basis for feeding all older people. The relation of calories to nutrients is described in the following experiment.

Diets of 100 white women, forty years of age and over, were measured over a period of time and the nutrient intakes estimated. With each reduction of calories, an equivalent reduction in protein, the "B" vitamins, iron, and calcium was found. When more than 2,000 calories were eaten each day, nutrients obtained were within the range of accepted standards. When only 1,000 calories were taken, all nutrient intakes were less than two-thirds of accepted standards with the exception of ascorbic acid and vitamin A which reflects the use of fruits and vegetables but not the staples of the diet. It is not suggested that sufficient nutrients cannot be crowded into 1,000 calories of food. However, few people achieve this happy result when they reduce their intake by "just eating less" although all too often this reduction is the way the patient interprets the advice which is given him by his physician.

A basic diet plan providing 1,000 calories is given in Table 9.1. This diet just meets the minimum daily dietary allowances of the Food and Nutrition Board. It does not, however, provide sweets, dressings, gravies, or alcohol and, if any of these are taken and substituted on an equicaloric basis for the food outlined in the table, one or more nutrients will be taken at less than desirable amounts. Calories may

TABLE 9.1

Basic Diet of 1000 Calories With Additions To Provide 1800 Calories

Food	Nutrient Provided by Diet		Standard Allowances
6 oz. meat, fish, or cheese	Calories	1000	Depends on age and activity
1 pt. low fat milk			
3 servings starches			
2 servings vegetables, green, yellow, or red	Protein, gm	76	70
	Calcium, gm	0.67	0.80
2 servings fruit, 1 high in ascorbic acid	Iron, mg	10	10
	Vitamin A, IU	3480	5000
3 pats fat	Thiamin, mg	1.36	1.50
	Riboflavin, mg	1.60	1.80
Added for 1800 Calories:	Ascorbic Acid, mg	103	75
1/7 apple pie			
3 pats fat	All standard allowances met with additions.		
2 tsp. blue cheese dressing			
3 tsp. sugar or jelly			

be added from almost any source the patient wishes, if the basic food pattern is included first, as demonstrated in the lower half of Table 9.1 which shows how the diet may be increased to provide 1,800 calories. Table 9.2 shows how these menu patterns can be converted into meals.

In the group of aging homemakers studied, the noon meal was the least well planned and consequently the lowest in the contribution of nutrients. Studies of the aged living in boarding or nursing homes suggest that the evening meal may be the poorest one of the day and that restlessness and the desire to get up very early may result from going to bed with an empty stomach. This may be further exaggerated if supper is served too early. A span of ten to twelve hours should elapse between breakfast and the last meal of the day.

Throughout adult life, men have certain advantages over women in maintaining good nutrition in that their food requirements are on the average about 25 per cent more than those of women, assuming equal activity. As pointed out above, the more food eaten the greater the probability that a complete diet will be obtained. This does not preclude undernutrition in the aging man but when it occurs, it is apt to be related to the loss of the wife who has been responsible for food preparation. Here are a few "rules of thumb" which can be applied to feeding the relatively healthy older person:

1. Calories can be controlled most effectively by leaving out fried food, rich desserts, heavy icings and candy, and large amounts of added fats. Oven-fried food in which added fat is small in amount is a good substitute. Fruit, milk, and eggs can be combined in simple pudding desserts that require only a little sugar. Vinegar, lemon, or tomato juice and spices can be

TABLE 9.2

MENUS PLANNED FROM DIETS DESCRIBED

Meal	1000 Calories	1800 Calories
Breakfast	Oatmeal, skim milk Applesauce Black coffee or tea	Oatmeal, skim milk 1 poached egg on 1 slice toast 1 pat butter Black coffee or tea
Mid-morning	Nothing	Applesauce
Luncheon	Casserole of: ½ cup cooked rice 2 oz. meat or tuna fish ¼ cup tomato puree ½ onion precooked with 1 tsp. oil top with crumbs from 1 soda cracker Half grapefruit Tea	Same casserole except: buttered crumbs from 2 crackers may be used Half grapefruit 1 tsp. sugar Tea
Mid-afternoon	Tea or black coffee	4 oz. skim milk
Dinner	4 oz. minute steak Buttered beets Green salad with lemon juice ½ dinner roll 1 tsp. butter 4 oz. junket made with skim milk and Sucaryl Coffee, if desired	4 oz. steak Buttered beets Green salad with 2 tsp. cheese dressing 2 dinner rolls 2 tsp. butter 1/7 of 9″ apple pie Coffee, if desired
Bedtime	6 oz. skim milk	6 oz. skim milk

added for flavoring in place of large amounts of fat. Two useful recipes are:

ZERO SALAD DRESSING

½ cup tomato juice
1 tbsp. onion (chopped)
2 tbsp. lemon juice or vinegar
1 tsp. Worcestershire sauce
salt and pepper

Chopped parsley or green pepper, horseradish or dry mustard, etc., may be added if desired. Combine ingredients in a jar with a tight-fitting top. Shake well before using.

WHIPPED DRY MILK TOPPING FOR DESSERTS

Makes 35 servings

6 oz. dry milk (see package for measure)
1½ cups ice water
⅓ cup lemon juice
⅓ cup sugar
1 tsp. vanilla
salt, to taste

Mix dry milk with ice water, whip to soft peak. Add lemon juice and continue beating. Add sugar gradually and beat to a stiff peak. Season. *Should be made within a half hour of serving.*

2. Dentures and missing teeth require cooked, soft food—more about that later.
3. Most older persons do well on smaller meals with a quick "pick-me-up" feeding between meals. Fruit, a beverage, or a simple sweet such as graham crackers or very simple cookies are a good choice. These between-meal snacks offer an additional opportunity for contacts with the group. Afternoon tea can be a festive occasion with the simplest of menus.
4. Older people, like children, eat better if the meal, instead of being eaten alone, is shared with others.
5. Family type service allows some choice in satisfaction of appetite. The situation may need some diplomatic monitoring to be sure that everyone eats well.
6. Help in eating should be unobtrusive but may be needed; i.e., cutting meat, buttering bread, etc.
7. Cookery and serving hints: Make maximum use of seasoning—taste acuity dulls with aging. Introduce occasional new foods or old foods cooked in new ways. See that every meal has at least one spot of bright color—a beet pickle, slice of cinnamon apple, a bright green leaf, or a highly colored vegetable. Eye appeal and taste appeal go hand in hand. Old-fashioned dishes such as roast beef hash or a good stew are a welcome change from meat, potatoes, and a vegetable. Use the oven to its maximum capacity. This not only results in good food but can be a saving of time and energy for the cook.
8. Meals and feedings should be spaced so that the night fast is never longer than ten–twelve hours.

MODIFIED DIETS

There was a time when modified diets for treatment of disease were "special" in the sense that the foods used bore no relation to the meals served for patients on regular diets. Much of this food, such as overcooked vegetables and nonnutritive food substitutes, was unpalatable and made special diets very burdensome. This need no longer be true. The patient who has a prescription for a modified diet may eat essentially the same food as his neighbor. There are two basic differences: first, the total amount of food may be limited; and second, the cookery may be modified, as in the omission of salt or in sieving and pureeing.

This discussion will be limited to the principles underlying some of the basic therapeutic diets in use, with suggestions as to where the nursing home administrator can go for detailed help. To attempt to be more specific at this point would be futile since, to a degree, each diet is tailored for the specific patient.

A most widely used modification of diet is that of consistency. When a food is cooked, it is softened in consistency. Grinding, sieving, and blending are all degrees of change in food from a solid to a liquid. If all spices are omitted in cookery, the soft-cooked or ground food is said to bland. Food modified in consistency is used for certain diseases of the intestinal tract; for instance, for a partial obstruction in the upper portion of the tract. A liquid or semiliquid passes an obstruction more easily than a solid. In the lower part of the intestine, food has been liquified by the digestive processes and the consistency as eaten is relatively unimportant.

The most frequent justification for a soft or semiliquid food for the aged is lack of strength to manage a plate of solid food or lack of teeth to masticate it. The latter is not always a good reason unless there is some limitation to swallowing, as most persons can eat solid food without teeth if it is tender, cut into small portions, or mashed with a fork.

A few foods should be avoided when soft consistencies are needed or when patients are very inactive: bran, onions, turnips, the cabbage family (except for the blossoms of cauliflower or broccoli), baked beans, food which is dipped in a batter and deep fried. Small seeds also are to be avoided (as in berries), though the pulp and juice may be used. In some bland, soft diets, fruit juices may need to be diluted and served in small portions several times a day. A good rule is to instruct the patient to take his juice at the end rather than at the beginning of the meal, but if it is part of the prescribed diet, it should not be omitted.

In practice, most elderly persons profit by division of the food into more than three meals, though the between-meal nourishments can be small in amount. For the patient with a restricted diet order, the between-meal nourishment cannot be added to food but must be a part of the entire day's diet plan.

The extreme modification in consistency is the formula diet which may be sipped through a polyethylene tube (but is usually given to a patient unable to eat). Any liquid food which will flow through the tube may be given as an emergency feeding. For a patient who needs rehabilitation or who may need to be fed for extended intervals by means of a tube, a planned formula is best, because it can be compounded to meet all the nutritional needs of the patient.

Formula diets are of two kinds:

1. *The diet based on some form of milk, including the products designed for infant feeding.* Carbohydrate in the form of glucose or dextrimaltose, fat (oil), or eggs, may be added for a complete food mixture. If eggs are used, a soft custard should be

prepared and then diluted to volume, rather than feeding a sick patient raw eggs and thus running a chance of salmonella-produced disease. A product containing eggs also should be passed through a fine sieve or coarse cheesecloth to eliminate lumps which might clog the tube.

2. *A diet of natural foods which is homogenized in a blender of the Waring type.* For best results, meat, fruit, and vegetables sold in individual jars for infant feeding are the best choice for blending. Full directions for preparing both types of formulas will be found in the materials listed on the source sheets included.

The second basic adjustment made in restricted diets is in the control of the amount of one or more of the food nutrients allowed the patient. These we designate as diets written to prescription. The diabetic diet or the diet restricted in fat or sodium are typical examples. There are several steps in the planning and preparation of such a diet. First, the doctor writes a prescription, usually in terms of calories, protein, fat, and carbohydrate. He may also designate what fraction of the total diet is to be served at each meal. The prescription, in turn, must be converted into a meal pattern or plan. Perhaps the doctor will do this for you or you may be able to enlist the help of a local dietitian. The diet plan is then made into menus by the staff of your institution, using a set of exchange lists such as that included with your illustrative material.

The exchange lists are based on the principle that many foods make similar contributions to the diet and a choice of food within a food group will allow for much greater variety and also allows you to use the same foods on your general menu for your special-diet patient. Just remember one basic rule: do not exchange foods between lists. For instance, extra bread or potato is not the same as orange juice or a green vegetable. If you have a patient who cannot or will not eat certain foods, the planning for this irregularity should be done in making up the meal pattern. Some prescriptions, however, do not lend themselves to indefinite adjustment.

MISCELLANEOUS INFORMATION

Useful publications:

Handbook of Experimental and Therapeutic Dietetics, M. A. Ohlson, ed. (Minneapolis: Burgess Publishing Co.). Price $4.00. Includes experimental and test diets and analyses for nutritive values of restricted diets. Emphasis is on "how to do," rather than "rule of thumb."

Simplified Diet Manual With Meal Patterns, Nutrition Service of the Iowa State Department of Health in cooperation with the Iowa Dietetic Association (Ames: Iowa State University Press, 1961). Price $2.50. Emphasis is on "rule of thumb." Designed for use by small hospitals without dietitian.

"The Regulation of Dietary Fat," Council on Foods and Nutrition of the American Medical Association, *Jour. Am. Med. Assn.,* August 4, 1962, p. 411.

The Special Diet Cook Book, M. Small (New York: Graystone Press). Basic recipes for cookery without salt, limited fats, etc.

Eat Well and Stay Well, Ancel and Margaret Keys (Garden City, N.Y.: Doubleday and Co., 1963). Low fat diets and recipes. Use of oils in cookery.

Source of sugar-free canned goods, and vegetables canned without added NaCl:

Chicago Dietetic Supply House, Inc.
1750 West Van Buren Street
Chicago 12, Illinois

Catalogs and price lists sent on request. This is a reliable firm and the products are more dependable than those sometimes found at the supermarket.

Useful addresses for obtaining late information on nutrition:

American Medical Association
535 North Dearborn Street
Chicago 10, Ill.

American Heart Association
44 East 23 Street
New York 10, N.Y.

National Academy of Sciences
Food and Nutrition Board
2101 Connecticut Avenue
Washington 25, D.C.

American Dietetic Association
620 North Mhichigan Avenue
Chicago 11, Ill.

Available (free) from the American Heart Association:

Your Mild Sodium-Restricted Diet
Your 1000 Milligram Sodium Diet (moderate sodium restriction)
Your 500 Milligram Sodium Diet (strict sodium restriction)
Planning Fat-Controlled Meals for Unrestricted Calories
Planning Fat-Controlled Meals for 1200 and 1800 Calories

Chapter 10

Meeting Dietary Needs

ANNABELLE L. MARTENEY, *M.S.*, WILLA A. SINGER, *B.S.*, DELORES A. BALTZ, *M.S.*, ROBERT A. SUTTON, *B.S.*, GERALDINE S. CLAYTON, *B.S.*

A. Menu Planning: Meals With Eye and Taste Appeal

ANNABELLE MARTENEY, *M.S.*

Equal parts of good food, good cooking, good health, good people to eat with, good places to eat, and good reasons for eating may be considered as conquerors of malnutrition.[1] Because older people tend to choose tea and toast which give only calories, there is need to be watchful and encouraging in feeding them. One of the beginning steps, in fact the foundation for good food in any food service, is the menu. When 10 to 15 per cent of the budget of a fifty-bed nursing home is spent for food, it is important that menus be *planned.*

Sometimes it is necessary to have menus planned and food prepared for nursing homes by people who are willing but who lack formal training. What suggestions can be given these people? Basically three things must be considered in planning menus: factors affecting the food service, tools to use in planning menus, and steps to use in actually writing a menu.

FACTORS AFFECTING FOOD SERVICE

Whenever anyone considers having good food for patients or residents he must first accept the responsibility for planning his own home or hospital. Briefly summarized, the factors to consider are the following: the needs of the patients, including the nutritional requirements; the desires of the patients (which are influenced by race, religion, tradition, and regional reflections); variety and appeal which include color, texture, flavor, shapes, and temperatures; seasonal factors, including holidays; availability of food, which is sometimes a seasonal factor but may also rely on transportation means within localities; the budget, which is indicated by management when the standard of service is determined (that is, whether it will be stew or steak!); personnel available and their individual skills; and the physical equipment and storage facilities.

Menu planning is not a routine procedure. It offers an opportunity to exercise imagination and ingenuity. It can be enjoyable and most certainly a challenge. A few tools assembled before tackling the task will be most helpful.

TOOLS TO USE IN PLANNING MENUS

A most important tool for the person doing the job is time—time freed from other duties and interruptions. It is best to have a work center equipped with pencils, a calendar with special holidays and fast days (if mixed religious groups are being served), and paper big enough for one week's menu. Menu forms are available from many sources or forms may be made by taking a large sheet of wrapping paper and ruling it for the number of meals and between-meal feedings.

When old menus are available they should be checked for food values, attractiveness, combinations, patient acceptance, cooks' work load, and cost. Also, tested recipes (with portion cost indicated) are helpful. When recipes are tested (standardized), the quantity of raw food needed may be easily determined. Having market quotations available will also be convenient.

It is wise to have a list of preferred dishes, as well as a guide for ways to use leftovers. Magazines with new recipes and with hints on how to improve products are worthwhile references, too.

Most important is the food guide that translates nutritional needs into prepared foods. The American Hospital Association's *Diet and Menu Guide*[2] gives information on how to plan menus using a standard meal pattern. Another reference, quite easily read and understood, is *Food Marketing Leaflet* #12.[3] One thing to remember in using a chart is that individual foods contain a variety of nutrients and there is an interdependence among groups, so direct substitution of groups is not possible. For example, milk is often thought of as a calcium source, but if another food is substituted for milk on that basis it must be remembered that milk is also important as a source of protein. Also, guides do not provide all the answers. However, if followed as directed, the meals planned from the guide are reasonably adequate nutritionally.

WRITING A MENU

Menus should be planned in advance, preferably for eight, three, or no less than one week at a time. Such planning eliminates repetition of foods and food combinations; it facilitates the purchase of supplies; and it is a basis for wise use of employees' time.

A menu may be one of two styles: a straight, planned menu or

TABLE 10.1

SUGGESTED BASIC FOOD PATTERN*

Foods To Include Daily	Quantity	Size of One Serving
I. Meat, Fish, Poultry, and Eggs		
Meat, poultry, or fish[1]	1 serving	3 to 4 ounces (edible portion)
Meat or alternate[2]	1 serving	1 ounce meat (or) ½ to ⅔ cup alternate
Egg	1 egg 3 or 4 times / week	1 egg
II. Milk, Cheese, and Ice Cream		
Milk	1 to 1½ pts.	1 glass (6 to 8 oz.)
III. Vegetables and Fruits		
Vegetable: one serving of a green, leafy, or yellow, and one other	2 servings	½ cup
Potato: white or sweet	1 or more servings	½ cup of 1 medium-sized potato
Fruit: one serving of citrus fruit or tomato or their juices, and one other	2 servings	½ cup; 4 oz. juice
IV. Breads and Cereals		
Whole-grain or enriched	4 or more servings	1 slice bread; ½ cup cooked cereal; (or) ⅔ cup ready-to-eat cereal
Butter or margarine	3 servings	2 level teaspoons

[1] Liver should be served once in two weeks.

[2] Meat or alternate includes either 1 oz. cheddar cheese, cottage cheese, meat, poultry, fish, peanut butter; ½ to ⅔ cup dried peas or beans, or 1 egg. These foods may be used singly or in combination with other foods.

* Source: *Diet and Menu Guide,* American Hospital Association, Chicago, Illinois, 1961.

its opposite, a selective menu (one where the patient may choose food items). Either style menu may be written as a cycle menu. The chief disadvantage of a cycle menu is that often it is written and forgotten. However, its advantages outweigh the disadvantages. Cycle menus are good when little supervision is possible. The employees can be instructed the first time around the cycle and there should be a carry-over of instructions when the menu is used again; time is saved since the menus are used periodically according to the length of the cycle and may be repeated on a seasonal basis.

It should be remembered that cycles may best be planned on either eight- or twelve-day periods to avoid the association of certain foods with particular weekdays, and the menu plan must be flexible in order that leftovers can be used wisely without lowering standards and so that fruits and vegetables can be changed with the season. Above all, it is important to observe the menus in connecting either weeks or days together to avoid needless repetition.

Regardless of the style menu used, some tricks of menu planning which might be helpful are:

1. Select the meat dishes or other main dishes for the noon meals (or heavy main meal) for each day, first.
2. Then select the main dish for the other meal.
3. Choose vegetables, salads, bread, and dessert to go with the meat or other main dish for noon; then evening.
4. Plan breakfast paying particular attention to including a citrus fruit or juice, if there is not one already on the menu for the other meals. Allow a selection of eggs, cereals, and beverages whenever possible.
5. Include at least two items on the general diet that can be used for soft diets and which, with minor change, can be used on other modified therapeutic diets. This modification may often be done with a change in the garnish, or by serving a fruit rather than a prepared dessert.
6. Include between-meal feedings in the planning. This is a good place to incorporate the juice for vitamin C, egg, or milk.
7. Include liver one time every two weeks. Find a way of preparing it that is acceptable to your situation. Many recipes are available. Creole liver is often most acceptable.
8. Every meal should include a protein dish such as egg, lean meat, poultry, fish, or cheese.
9. Try a new dish once a week.
10. If adults reject milk, add nonfat milk solids in cookery.
11. Remember the number to be fed. Some food products are not the same when the preparation is for a large group.
12. Take into consideration that the appetites of men and women differ not only in size of portions, but in the kinds of foods liked.

To help with future menu planning, make a menu file. It would be wise to record the reaction of those eating the food as planned and prepared, the difficulty or ease of preparation, and the cost of the portion, either on the menus or on individual recipes. A cycle may be prepared from menus saved over a period of time. Also, menus on permanent file are helpful to standard-setting agencies in determining the adequacy of meals served.

SUMMARY

In menu planning accept as a goal that the meals be nutritionally adequate, and if the food is not eaten the food service management has failed. It's the acceptability, or what's eaten, that counts! It has been said that a patient can compare only two things with his home: his food and his bed.

Even though a budget is limited, and there are few employees or modern conveniences, any nursing home can have palatable and nutritious food provided menus are planned to meet the needs of that particular home.

RECIPES FROM FILES OF MAIN KITCHEN NUTRITION DEPARTMENT, UNIVERSITY HOSPITAL, IOWA CITY

CREOLE LIVER

Ingredients	*Adapted to*		
	25	*50*	*100*
Liver	6 lb.	12½ lb.	25 lb.
Onion	½ lb.	1 lb.	2 lb.
Fat	¼ lb.	½ lb.	1 lb.
Catsup	3 cups	6 cups	12 cups
Tomatoes, canned	3 cups	6 cups	12 cups
Peppers	¼ lb.	½ lb.	1 lb.
Worcestershire sauce	½ tbsp.	1 tbsp.	2 tbsp.
Salt	2½ tbsp.	5 tbsp.	10 tbsp.
Pepper	½ tsp.	1 tsp.	2 tsp.
Flour for dredging			

Method:

1. Dredge liver in flour and brown in skillet or on grill. Place in deep casserole or roaster. (Pans must be deep enough to add creole mixture.) Set aside.
2. Brown onions in fat. Add all other ingredients to the onions, except liver, and simmer 10–15 minutes.
3. Pour simmered mixture on top of liver.
4. Cook in oven approximately 1½ hours at 350°.

CRUMB COOKIES

Ingredients	*Adapted to*		
	30	*60*	*120*
Oleo	½ lb.	1 lb.	2 lb.
Brown sugar, firmly packed*	¾ cup	1½ cups	3 cups
Eggs, whole	3	6	1 doz.
Flour, sifted	4⅛ cups	7⅛ cups	14¼ cups
Baking powder	4 tsp.	2½ tbsp.	5 tbsp.
Salt	¼ tsp.	¾ tsp.	1½ tsp.
Milk	1½ cups	3 cups	1½ qt.
Crumbs	1¼ lb.	2½ lb.	5 lb.
Raisins	¼ lb.	½ lb.	1 lb.
Vanilla	1 tsp.	2 tsp.	4 tsp.

* If using cake and frosting for crumbs cut sugar in half.

Method:

1. Cream shortening and sugar. Add slightly beaten eggs.
2. Sift flour, baking powder, and salt together.
3. Add dry ingredients and milk alternately to the creamed mixture.
4. Add crumbs, raisins, and vanilla.
5. Drop on oiled baking sheet.
6. Bake at 350° 10–12 minutes.

B. Food Preparation: Controlling Quality and Cost in the Kitchen

WILLA A. SINGER, *B.S.*

The basic goals to be considered in achieving quality food include conserving the nutritive value of the food; improving the digestibility; developing and enhancing flavor; increasing (or at least retaining) the attractiveness of original color, form, and texture; and keeping the food free from injurious organisms and substances. Some may prefer to think of these as the three "T's" of proper food preparation: training, timing, and tasting. Proper training of employees and the correct timing of food production are essential to serving foods as soon after preparation as possible. Nothing is so inviting as freshly cooked meat or pie still warm from the oven. Tasting during production is important also; it may save money and prevent future problems. Foods should be sampled prior to service to check for correct temperature, adequate seasoning, and proper consistency.

Foods need to be basically good to start with, for one poor-quality ingredient may ruin an entire product. Also, the purpose for which the food is intended needs to be considered, since a lesser grade may be acceptable in many dishes, providing it meets nutritive requirements.

Many institutions today are relying on standardized recipes to take the guesswork out of cooking. A standardized recipe is one tested a number of times and found to be consistently satisfactory both in quality and yield. Standardizing recipes permits serving appetizing food with a minimum loss of nutritive value; it improves the control of yields (fewer leftovers); and it encourages greater labor efficiency. This system also is a means of determining more exactly the amount of food to purchase thus controlling cost. The cooperation and interest of everyone concerned, along with good supervision, is needed before beginning to standardize recipes, or even successfully continuing to use such a system. However, once recipes have been tested and proven, the reliance on one person to prepare a certain dish is eliminated and anyone should be able to prepare the same standard-quality product.

Recipes should be standardized to meet the needs of the institution, according to the quantities usually prepared. Various sources of recipes are available, but a word of warning in regard to household-sized recipes is in order. A household-sized recipe multiplied too many times cannot be counted on to give a desirable quantity product since the relative proportions of ingredients may be incorrect, the mixing time too short, the yield incorrect, or the length of cooking time inaccurate because larger quantities require longer to heat. Elaborate equipment is unnecessary; however, good scales, correct measuring and mixing tools, and ovens with correct temperature regulators are needed.

In developing a standardized recipe file, specific menu items should be selected and scheduled for production. New recipes may be used, in which case a small-quantity recipe from a reliable source should be tried first, or, if working with recipes which are already in use, evaluations should be made on small quantities since they represent a more reliable source of information. If interest is centered on putting a present unwritten recipe into written form, then the cooking should be observed and quantities and directions recorded in order to establish a trial form of the recipe. A product should be prepared exactly according to the recipe directions, and the evaluation based on such factors as flavor, appearance, ease of preparation, availability of ingredients, cost, and correct yield (within ten servings plus or minus of anticipated yield). The opinions of supervisors, cooks, and patients should be considered, and the recipe adjusted on this small-quantity basis before increasing to larger quantities. If a successful reproduction is achieved at twenty-five servings, the recipe can generally be increased further with little difficulty. When the recipe is satisfactorily produced in quantity, the final recipe may be written and added to a permanent file.

Any or all of the three main forms of recording recipes may be used in a recipe file. The standard form lists all ingredients first, followed by the Method, given in paragraphs or steps. This form is especially good for recipes calling for many ingredients.

Another recipe style, called the action form, combines narrative action with listed ingredients. This form is fairly easy to follow; however, it takes more space on a card and is difficult to arrange economically or attractively on paper, especially if many yield columns are desirable.

A third form, the narrative form, includes the amounts of ingredients along with the method. This is especially good for short or spoken recipes, or in those consisting of few ingredients but a more complex method. This is often used to state various procedures.

Recipes should be written so they will be simple and clear, accurate, and complete in essentials. When the quality of a dish depends on special ingredients or an exact procedure, the recipe should include this information. The ingredients should be listed in the order used, and level measurements used for all items. Abbreviations should be used only when necessary to conserve space. It is helpful to state the amounts of ingredients in the easiest and simplest measurements (1/4 cup instead of 4 tablespoons). Except in cases where another measure would be more accurate and convenient, it is better to state the quantity in terms of weights. When an ingredient is modified the exact measurement should be stated. That is, 2 cups sifted flour, not 2 cups flour, sifted. Descriptive word pictures are helpful, such as chill until syrupy, or beat until foamy, and the method should include the various mixing times necessary, temperature for cooking, and pan sizes.

The recipe file should be arranged according to food categories, and the recipe card should include the title of the recipe, the category under which it is filed, various yields, the date completed or revised, and a space for costing the recipe. Once a standardized recipe file is established, it should be periodically revised and recosted due to changes in personnel, equipment, costs, menus, and new food products.

In the steps toward quality food preparation the person's psychological as well as nutritional needs need to be considered. Food needs to be pleasing both to the eye and to the palate. This can be accomplished by a variety in color, flavor, and texture, and by remembering that good cooking doesn't mean the same to all people.

One of the greatest offenses to food preparation is overcooking of foods. When the preparation of food involves cooking, destruction of vitamins and minerals occurs. The conditions of preparation best suited to the retention of color, flavor, aroma, and texture tend also to preserve the nutrient value. The quick cooking of vegetables and fruits with minimum exposure to air results in the least loss of nutrients, and cooking in small quantities (5 lb. or 10 lb. lots) permits better heat penetration throughout and thus prevents overcooking. Vegetables are cooked adequately the minute they are tender, but they continue to cook if left standing in the container prior to service. Cooking in an excess amount of water increases nutrient losses. Flavor losses occur with overcooking because of the volatile substances which are driven off or changed. Both quality and money (due to food shrinkage) are lost when meats are overcooked. A temperature of 325° should be adequate for roasting meats, since protein items generally need lower temperatures and longer cooking times.

Foods should be prepared so that the original form is maintained, or some other form at least as pleasing is produced. Texture is closely associated with form also, and where alterations of form and texture are produced, the food preparation should be suited to producing the qualities considered as desirable and characteristic of a standard product. Variety may be added by preparing foods in a variety of shapes by dicing, shredding, slicing, molding into balls, or cutting wedges, blocks, or strips. Some of the typical food service pitfalls (which should be avoided at all cost) include salad ingredients so finely shredded that they lose their identity; creamed dishes of a pasty consistency; the cheese dish that strings; cookies too brittle for easy handling; vegetables cut into too large chunks; potatoes so large that they appear to dominate the plate; and "scrappy-looking" meat.

Tasty, well-seasoned foods are also important for quality food. The sense of taste dulls with age, hence older people generally do want sharp, definite flavors. Unless an individual's diet order restricts seasonings, don't assume all their food needs to be bland. Generally, if the person likes a food, his digestive tract will be able to handle it, but judgment needs to be exercised in the use of strong-flavored vegetables, melon, and certain other so-called "gas formers."

For the older person foods often need to be modified either because of diet or dentition. However, it is best to change the form only enough to meet each individual's needs, and avoid cooking, grinding, or pureeing until the food has lost all of its identity. By planning ahead it may be possible to simplify food production, and allow the same menu item to be served on a wide variety of diets. This may be done by omitting the gravy on some diets; by removing part of the product before adding salt; omitting fruit or nuts in part of the dessert, ice cream, or sauce; omitting irritating seasonings in casserole dishes; or by offering a juice in place of a salad or vegetable at a meal.

Nonfat, dry-milk solids may be used in various recipes in place of milk, both as a means of cutting food costs, and to improve the nutrient value of the food. Dry-milk powder basically may be substituted in any recipe that calls for milk, the type of recipe determining whether it is to be added as powder with the dry ingredients and then the water added, or whether it is to be reconstituted and used as milk. The nutrient value may be increased by either adding the powder as an extra item in the food, or by substituting for milk at one and one-half times the normal strength.

The use of garnishes to perk up dishes may be rewarding by bringing about added acceptance and interest in food. These do not need to be costly additions, for hundreds of ideas are available from the use of common fruits and vegetables and some protein items. Diversity in form, imagination, and variety are the key elements necessary. Various methods of preparing and cooking of the same food item also produce interesting variety.

Next, but certainly not least among the goals of good food service, is sanitation. Sanitation refers to the prevention of diseases by eliminating, or controlling, the environmental factors which form links in the chain of transmission. Proper sanitation is basic to high standards of food service, and it does not just happen—it requires the constant work and cooperation of everyone involved. The health and personal hygiene of employees, along with their food-handling techniques, need to be considered. The source of supply of food as well as proper refrigeration and storage after receiving, are important. An efficient dishwashing operation, along with general good housekeeping techniques, and equipment which can be easily cleaned, are all involved in an efficient sanitation program. The danger of contamination during food preparation may be lessened by eliminating "extra care" items (custards, puddings, cream products) between June 1 and September 15; by holding food at temperatures either below 45° F. or above 145° F. to prevent multiplication of any bacteria; by avoiding holding food for a long time prior to service; and by using excess processed food as soon as possible (in leftovers). Sanitation must be thought of as a way of life in order to be successful in a food service.

C. Food Service in the Dining Room and at the Bedside

DELORES A. BALTZ, *M.S.*

The service of food is important because food nourishes psychologically as well as physically. Food has been equated with love and speaks of your interest in your residents. Many elderly persons may come to you malnourished, not because of lack of food but because of loneliness and sorrow. They must be encouraged to eat by attractive food service.

The times of food service are important. Meals should be scheduled so that there is at least a ten-hour period between breakfast and the evening meal, leaving no more than fourteen hours between the evening meal and breakfast. It is recommended that the large meal be served in the evening because of the time lapse until breakfast, and because most people are used to this. It is now recognized that hunger during the night will cause more insomnia than indigestion from the larger evening meal. If meals over a ten-hour period, or serving dinner in the evening causes difficulty in scheduling kitchen personnel, it is recommended that the cook be scheduled over the luncheon and dinner meals, not because breakfast is any less important, but because the preparation of standard breakfast items can be accomplished by a less-skilled worker. Part-time help, especially high school students, can be used effectively.

Because of waning appetites in the elderly the food should be attractively arranged and well garnished. Although small amounts should be served initially, second helpings should be available and these should be encouragingly offered because many elderly people will not ask for more. The china, glassware, and flatware used should be functional but of a material, size, pattern, and color that will enhance the appearance of the food.

All residents who are able and willing (and some not so willing) should be served in the dining room. Mealtimes are more sacred to older generations than to younger generations. They are social times which break the monotony of a dull day. Socialization brings people out of themselves and their troubles and encourages eating by dispelling moodiness and despondency. Food tastes better and most residents will eat more, and in a better variety, in the dining room. Dining room service avoids cold food and delayed trays and facilitates the offering of choices and seconds.

From the standpoint of the administrator, dining room service is the more economical method. Surveys have shown that food waste in dining rooms is only one-half that of tray service. The fewer personnel required means a real saving in labor costs. A less tangible benefit derived is that critical eaters will put less emphasis on food, and the attitude of satisfaction with the better food service carries over to other areas.

The dining room should be cheerful and well lighted. Small tables, seating four to six persons, are more homelike and less institutional. Some tables should be high enough so that wheelchairs slide under allowing the patient to be close enough to the table for comfortable eating. The dining room should be large enough and arranged in such a way that there is enough space between tables for easy maneuverability of wheelchairs. Between meals, the dining room need not be wasted space but can be used for a recreation area, an employee lounge area, or for meetings.

Dining room service may be by either family style (portions selected at table) or by plate arrangement (portions served from the kitchen). Family style is the most popular because it allows the resident to make his own choice of food and size of serving, the food stays hotter, and second helpings are more easily available. Food waste is held to a minimum with this type of service. If plate service is used, portions should be small and well defined. Some method should be devised (perhaps a readily available cart), for providing second servings, beverages, and condiments.

One of the best methods for evaluating service in the dining room is to assign the staff, on a rotating basis, to eat with the residents and to make recommendations for improvements in the service.

There will always be some residents who are unable to come to the dining room. The same principles of good food service outlined above apply to trays served the patient at the bedside. These principles are of even more importance here. The tray should be attractively arranged, portions well defined, with garnishes added for interest and color. The attitude of the person serving the tray is of utmost importance. A pleasant, helpful, leisurely approach is best. A remark or facial expression showing dislike of the food by the person serving is often enough to prevent the patient's even tasting it. The tray must be firmly supported to prevent upsetting.

Positioning at a comfortable height will allow the patient to eat more before tiring. The muscular weakness caused by the inactivity of these bedfast patients requires that their food be cut into bite-sized pieces and beverages poured with sugar, etc., added. This should be done at the bedside to allow the patient the pleasure of seeing the food before it is cut up and to retain as much as possible of the original temperature and flavor. If the patient is capable of sitting up at all it is well worth the extra effort to get him out of bed so that he can eat at a small table in his room. The vertical position while eating will not only improve his appetite but will improve his digestion also.

Because of lagging appetites and physical disability, many senior citizens cannot eat enough at mealtimes to satisfy their nutrient requirements, and nourishment between meals is a necessity. The foods served at these times should be carefully planned to complement the daily menu. Emphasize nourishing liquids because most oldsters do not drink enough fluids. Again, these must be routinely offered; do not wait for them to be requested. An attractive nourishment cart, set up with choices of beverages, cookies, crackers, etc., could be circulated. For ambulatory patients a "coffee break" table in the dining room could be used.

Since most of the patrons in nursing homes must eat all their meals at the home, variety is needed to prevent eating from becoming just a boring routine. Sunday is perhaps the worst day to be separated from family and friends and something special is especially appreciated to look forward to. But celebrations should not be limited to Sunday, lest these, too, become routine. If Sunday is visitor day and the time during the week lags, a "dress up" dinner one night a week with tablecloths and entertainment may be the answer. With a little imagination, a reason for celebrating can be found for any day of the year. Special menus and decorations in the dining room need not be elaborate to carry out a party theme. Birthdays are usually celebrated with cake and song, but if space allows perhaps the resident could invite family or friends to be his guests on his birthday. He might even be consulted to help write the menu for his special meal.

For a change of pace, buffet service can be employed with beverages and desserts served after seating. If a special current event is being televised, trays might be carried to the TV room. Picnics are a pleasant change after eating so many meals indoors, but these should not be limited to the evening hours. During the summer months breakfast cookouts, while it is still cool outdoors, can start the day off on a holiday note. Like children, oldsters love a surprise, so, occasionally, complete secrecy about a special meal is a real thrill for them.

Special meals should not be for those in the dining room only.

Holiday themes can be carried out on trays with the use of tray covers and favors. Occasionally, a bedfast patient might have a "guest" in his room for a meal. This could be another resident or a visiting relative or friend.

D. Food Service Administration: Controlling Quality and Cost at the Desk

ROBERT A. SUTTON, *B.S.*

Food operations, no matter whether they are in public restaurants, hotels, hospitals, retirement homes, or nursing homes, have basically the same functions; i.e., purchasing, receiving, storage, preparation, and service. The extent to which these functions are carried out wisely and efficiently measures the success or failure of every type of operation. It is obvious that problems will differ in scope and perspective in the different areas, but nursing homes, still in their infancy compared to the other operations, can learn much from the experience of the restauranteur or hotel manager.

Proper purchasing is a procedure that provides an operation with the products most suited to its needs at the most economical price possible. It is with the elements of this definition that this paper is most concerned. What are the best procedures? What merchandise is best suited and how can it be so determined? How and when can this merchandise be purchased most economically?

It is recognized that only a few nursing homes will be in the position of having a food buyer whose duties will be exclusively devoted to this area. Rather, the administrator, who will have multiresponsibilities and duties, will be the person responsible not only for maintaining the proper food-cost figure, but also for purchasing the food to meet the operation's needs.

The administrator should gain a working knowledge of such kitchen production problems as what is involved when purchasing wholesale cuts of meat, rather than portion-sized cuts. He should be able to tell the dealer why the roast was poor and he should know why water-pack or light-syrup–pack fruits are best for salads. The administrator should be able to tell the kitchen staff why it is best to roast for a longer time and at a lower temperature. He should be ready to correct the cooks on improper slicing, serving, and the storage of leftovers. If the operation uses steam tables, he should know that the Blue Lake green bean will stand up much better than the common variety of green bean.

The administrator will need to be well versed in market trends. He should know how stock prices in Chicago today will affect local markets the following week. He should be able to judge whether a fair price, based on current market reports, was quoted on produce by his local dealer.

Three basic purchasing procedures are available:

1. Open market purchasing. This is used by the majority of of all operations. It is seeking prices from one or more purveyors and accepting those terms that are the most advantageous to the buyer, all elements of price, quality, yield, and service having been considered.
2. Sealed bid purchasing. The name is self-explanatory. It is customarily thought that this is suited to larger operations; however, any size working unit can profit from this method. You can tally your past records for a given period on certain items, such as dairy products and bread, and ask for bids on the same amounts for the future. It may be suprising to find how competitive some companies will become to gain or retain your business.
3. Futures and contract purchasing. This method is used but little today. It is a speculative forecast where you purchase in large quantities, anticipating price increases. Buyers might better concentrate on operations and leave the speculating to the jobbers.

The major sources of supply usually available are:

1. Wholesale food houses. These constitute the commonest purveyors of food to most operations. Briefly, they perform the service function of jobbers, accumulating varieties of merchandise from many sources and offering them for demand sale.
2. Manufacturers and packers. Many sources, such as ice cream plants, bakeries, coffee salesmen, and meat packers, sell directly to the user. Some buyers try to eliminate the middleman by purchasing directly from the manufacturer for other food items. This is ideal when prices are better than the local markets; however, many believe that just because they buy direct, prices will be lower. This is not always true and it is best to obtain prices from the wholesale houses.
3. Local farmers and producers. Fortunately, in some states we are close to markets and we can receive daily supplies of fresh fruits and vegetables in season. However, it is the wise buyer who will be comparing the Chicago market with local prices.
4. Municipal markets. Usually these are found in the larger cities. These markets are basically the same as the above.
5. Cooperative associations. In the last fifteen years these organizations have become increasingly important in the wholesale field. They consist of many producers (usually farm and dairy products) who combine for the benefits gained through central and large-scale distribution and selling.
6. Retail food stores. Except for emergency use, these markets

are not recommended. They are geared to sell to the retail trade, and even though some offer price reductions, the food buyer can usually obtain better prices elsewhere.

Most states and the federal government have set up standards and specifications concerning packs, grades, and varieties. The wise food buyer will recognize the value of these standards in obtaining quality and use them wherever practical. It must be emphasized, however, that written standards and specifications cannot be a substitute for a buyer's skill. Specifications should be written on all products usually purchased. Information for complete and detailed writing should be based on experience as well as government information.

The following is a well-written specification as taken from the *Manual of Specifications for Canned Fruits and Vegetables* by the American Hospital Association.

ORANGE JUICE SWEETENED OR UNSWEETENED * U.S. GRADE A (FANCY) canned orange juice to be undiluted, unfermented juice from matured fresh oranges. The juice to possess a bright yellow to yellow-orange color typical of freshly extracted juice and to be free from traces of browning due to scorching, oxidation, caramelization or other causes; to be practically free from defects, to show no coagulation and there may be present not more than .030 per cent by volume of recoverable oil, and shall contain no noticeable particles of membrane, core, skin, seeds and seed particles, similar substances or other defects; to possess a fine, distinct, normal orange juice flavor, free from traces of scorching, caramelization, oxidation or terpene, and shall test not less than 10.5 degrees Brix, and contain not less than 0.75 gm. nor more than 1.4 gm. acid calculated as anhydrous citric per 100 milliliters of juice. Total score not less than 85 points.

Specify Style as Sweetened or Unsweetened: Canned orange juice may be considered "Sweetened" if sugar has been added and the juice tests not less than 13.5 degrees Brix.

Approximate Net Measure: No. 2 tin—1 pint 2 fluid oz.; *No. 3 cyl.—1 quart 14 fluid oz.; *No. 10—3 quarts.

Specification: U.S. Grade A (Fancy); Unsweetened; Minimum Brix cut out 10.5 degrees; No. 2 tin; No. 3 cyl.; No. 10.

It is common practice for many operations to allow deliverymen to supply to a standing order or to a par stock. This not only leaves the operation open to the dishonest deliveryman, but also overloads the storage facilities and creates a larger inventory that necessitates increased handling, and, therefore, higher labor cost.

The food buyer has a responsibility to see that the merchandise ordered is the merchandise received. Whether you check all deliveries or spot-check occasionally, you are going to make your purveyors aware that you do not plan to be a disposal for goods not wanted by others. You should appoint one member of your staff to do all the receiving. This person should be able to recognize different grades and to follow your written specifications for goods ordered.

A guide to the food buyer as to his proper purchasing can be measured, in part, with a food-cost accounting system, or food-cost control as it is generally called. Whether the operation is large or small some accounting controls should be kept. The purpose of a food-cost control system is to assist management to keep the cost of food consumed at the lowest possible point, consistent with management's policy as to quality and size of portions.

While a food-cost system may, and often does, bring out the fact that portions are unreasonably large, it is not the aim of such a system to reduce cost by reducing portions. Above all, a food-control system should never be allowed to go as far as to cause any lowering of the quality of the materials used.

The general effect of the installation of a food-cost control system often results in reducing the cost to a considerable extent, but the system cannot of itself produce the desired result any more than a good road map can drive an automobile. Food-cost control does, however, give the timely warning as soon as the cost turns in the wrong direction, and it points out where and how to turn for the right road. It is then up to the management to take the necessary action.

The essential requisites of such a system can be summed up briefly in three points:

1. It must be practical—that is, it must not interfere with the working routine of the kitchen.
2. It must give sufficient detailed information on which to base corrective measures.
3. The cost must be considerably less than the savings it affects.

No report on a food operation is of great consequence unless it is made available to management in time to permit corrective measures where necessary. A simplified system is where all goods issued from storage areas are recorded daily. They are priced and then divided by the number of meals served. This, of course, will show both meal cost and total daily food cost. This system will be subjected to many variables, such as not recording spices used, flour used as a thickening agent, and condiments used. These items are not usually recorded daily except when issued from storage in the bulk form.

The monthly report summarizes the daily reports and is used to gain a better picture of the operation over a longer period. Inventories need to be taken, both in storage areas and production areas. Sale of by-products (grease, bones, etc.) are entered; credit for returned merchandise is recorded; and detergents, paper supplies, and other expendable items are recorded. The semiannual or annual reports are the compilation of the monthly reports.

Some operations find it beneficial to precontrol or precost their food department. This is the procedure of forecasting the number of meals to be served, then costing the menu accordingly.

Three fundamental procedures must be set up before precontrol can be effective. The first is the establishment of the average usable yields from the raw foods as purchased. This is accomplished by testing the specified grade, weight, size, or count of purchased foods for the percentage of trim and shrinkage loss in preparing the item for use. These tests reveal much, including the economical grade and size to be purchased.

The second procedure is the establishment of standardized recipes and portion sizes. The preparation of all food selections requiring a blending of ingredients (such as for extended dishes), should be standardized by measurement and the costs determined. Whenever the selection is offered, the patient is assured a uniform product and management is assured a uniform cost.

The last procedure to be established for the precost function is an analysis of the consumption of all items offered. Thus, a file should be kept on the daily menu as to what is the best and the least acceptable of the items offered. This information should be used for future menu-planning decisions.

It must be remembered that for any accounting system that no one "best" system exists for every operation. It needs to be tailored to fit your operation. An accounting system is never a substitute for supervision—direct supervision is still necessary. It should be remembered also that all systems should be reviewed periodically by management.

E. Food Service Administration: Personnel Management

GERALDINE S. CLAYTON, *B.S.*

In any business, hospital, restaurant, nursing home, or retirement home, it is necessary to set up standards of procedure and to keep accurate records of pay schedules, promotions or reference, hiring, and discharging.

List the number of people working as nurse, nurse's aide, cook, cook's helper, diet worker, waiter, gardener, etc. Draw up a full job description for each job from the hour the worker reports for duty until he signs out. Sign-in and sign-out is a matter of record for pay purposes.

Job descriptions are not hard and fast rules; they serve as a guide and check to the worker and can be changed. In a kitchen the number of workers needed depends upon many things: the number of people to be served; how they are served, in rooms or in a dining room; the kind of equipment used; labor-saving equipment; frozen and canned foods, or fresh foods which require longer preparation.

A job description justifies the job. In case personnel is reduced, items can be studied, and changes made accordingly.

A supervisor is necessary as a coordinator between management and workers. In a small kitchen this may be the owner. A supervisor's duties are:

ADMINISTRATIVE

1. Schedules all personnel, working hours, holidays, vacations. Schedules should show definite days off. A day off is necessary, no matter how small the establishment. The individual needs rest and a change of scene. It prevents the feeling that the place can't operate without him.

   If workers are on an 8-hour schedule, their duty hours may be staggered: cook comes in early, 5:30 A.M. until 2:00 P.M.; helper at 6:00 A.M. until 2:30 P.M., depending on number to be served; others at 10:30 A.M. until 7:00 P.M. The full crew is on through the noon meal, and until extra cleaning and supper preparations are accomplished. The serving of supper may be left for a minimum crew with the help of a high school boy or girl who is paid by the hour (from 5:00 P.M. until 7:00 P.M.) to serve and wash dishes.
2. Interviews, hires, and fires. When hiring some things to be considered are: Where does applicant live? Will he be able to get to work in all weather? Will family responsibilities present problems (preschool children, and the like)? Age, physical health, any chronic illness? Experience? Etc.
3. Keeps all records relative to holidays, sick leave, etc. Keep rating cards on each employee for recommendations, promotions.
4. Trains new employees.
5. Works varied hours to cover the whole day.

ORGANIZATIONAL

1. The food-service supervisor must have a working knowledge of diet therapy in order to work in absence of the dietitian or with a part-time dietitian.
2. She (most generally, food supervisors are women) should be a communication center. All directions or orders go through her from management to worker. Likewise, complaints from workers go through her to management.
3. She must be familiar with aseptic techniques (isolation, uniforms, caps, etc.), as well as food storage, the proper use of leftovers, etc.
4. She must be familiar with the job of every employee.
5. She must know where to order foods (baked food, ice cream, meats, etc.)

6. She must know how to check deliveries for proper weights, etc.
7. She must know how to operate all equipment, and to check the care and maintenance of same (mixers, toasters, dishwashers, etc.) She must know how to make out the cook's sheet. She must be fair and consistent.

SANITATION

1. All food-service workers must wear a clean uniform daily, and a hair net or a cap. Boys wear clean white jackets if working part time. Uniforms may be furnished and laundered in the establishment or, if working in a small unit, an employee may furnish her own.

SAMPLE OF RATING CARD

Name ______________________ Classification ______________

Began Work ________________ Termination Date ____________

(a) Quantity of work produced
(b) Quality of work produced
(c) Adaptability
(d) Initiative (Can he take or accept responsibility?)
(e) Manner of performance (adept at work, quiet and respectful, language seemly, etc.)
(f) Attitude
(g) Other

These cards should be checked at least once a year, and the person rated by the supervisor. If the worker is not up to par or any change is shown, the supervisor should call him in to discuss the matter.

EXAMPLE OF JOB DESCRIPTION

25 trays. Only cook and helper on duty. Cook's helper—6:30 a.m.–3:00 p.m.

6:30 Finish setting up cold trays, pour juice, etc.
7:00 Put on milk, butter, jelly, and make toast, load hot cart.
7:30 Take hot cart to ward, help serve trays, pick up trays.
8:00 Strip trays and wash dishes.
8:45 Reset trays for dinner, clean and refill salt and pepper shakers and sugar bowls, if used. Put away food deliveries.
9:15 Coffee break.
9:30 Help cook prepare vegetables and make salads.
11:00 Eat lunch.
11:30 Set up cold trays, salad, dessert, milk, butter, etc.
12:00 Take hot cart to ward, help with serving trays.
12:30 Help pick up trays, wash dishes, reset trays.
1:45 Clean and arrange storeroom neatly, wipe up floor.
2:15 Clean refrigerator, check all leftover food, discard if 24 hours old.
3:00 Sign out.

FOOTNOTES

1. Monroe, R. T., M.D., *Diseases in Old Age.* Cambridge, Mass.: Harvard University Press, 1951.
2. *Diet and Menu Guide.* American Hospital Association, Chicago, Illinois, 1961.
3. *Food Marketing Leaflet* #12. New York State Extension Service, Cornell University, Ithaca, N.Y., 1961.

ADDITIONAL READINGS

4. Hospital Food Notes, "Dietary Consultant Helps Iowa Hospitals Plan Practical and Pleasing Menus." *Hospitals,* 37:7:65, 1963.
5. Smith, Charlotte E., "Working Toward Food Service Goals for Nursing Homes." *Hospitals,* 36:2:91, 1962.
6. "Old Folks in Homes." *Institutions,* 52:4:67, 1963.
7. Nyhus, Delores L., "For the Long-Term Patient: Food Plus Understanding." *Hospitals,* 36:6:71, 1962.
8. Hospital Food Notes, "How Nursing Homes Plan Menus." *Hospitals,* 36:6:79, 1962.
9. *Menu Planning, Food Buying for Small Hospitals and Nursing Homes.* School of Home Economics, University of Alabama, 1960.

Part Five

RECREATION AND GROUP PROCEDURES

Chapter 11

The Role of Recreation

JANET R. MacLEAN, *Dr. Recreation*

Much has been said about recreation and the recreation needs of the elderly in the last few years. Let us consider first, however, the subject of recreation itself.

Even the dictionary doesn't always have the right answer when words are used among people with different experience backgrounds. Two examples illustrate my point. If the female readers of this book were called a "vision" today by a member of the opposite sex, I'm sure they would react quite differently from the way they would respond if they were called a "sight"—yet Webster's "unabridged" gives both terms like definitions. A friend of mine had similar problems with his six-year-old son. Standing on a high ladder, trying to hang the latest purchase for his art collection, he asked Karl to get him a screwdriver. After a lengthy interval, Karl returned with the message, "Sorry, Dad, I found the orange juice but we're out of vodka." We might recall the famous quotation of the naval commander who in the heat of battle shouted bravely, "We have not yet *begun* to fight." A wounded sailor lying near him on the deck moaned, "Somebody's always not getting the word."

All of us who work with the elderly should "get the word," and that word is recreation. The word recreation has been greatly misused and misunderstood. To some it connotes children at play; to others, a banner to be waved against social ills; to some, meaningless frivolity; to others, a charity for the underprivileged; to still others, creative meaningful activity. In fact, recreation is such a highly personal experience that it almost defies concrete definition.

If I were to ask lay and professional persons to explain the term, I might receive a variety of responses, each rooted in a personal philosophy or conditioned by past experience. Although definitions vary, most of them describe recreation as activity as opposed to idleness; it is done in leisure; a person participates because he wants to do so; the satisfactions are immediate, enjoyable, and inherent in the activity. Here are two definitions, similar, yet with slightly different emphases.

The first is my own: "Recreation is any enjoyable leisure experience in which the participant voluntarily engages and from which he receives immediate satisfactions." The second is Paul Douglass' descriptive capsule which captures the essence of recreation as "unhurried, pleasurable living among man's spontaneous and educated enthusiasms." Such definitions of recreation are broad enough to include many experiences. No specific activity may be designated as recreation; recreation is person-centered. Your attitude toward the activity is all important. Recreation may include reading a book, playing football, attending a symphony, or baby-sitting. The potential of recreation for creative, satisfying enriched living in increased leisure is limitless.

Why get all excited now in the 1960's about recreation? Why has society shown concern? Isn't what a person does for recreation his own business? Why all the fuss now? How does it happen that a whole new profession has evolved to serve the recreation needs of young and old in our generation? Change is an eternal phenomenon in human history, but the twentieth century has brought changes at such an accelerated pace that the lives of all have been revolutionized.

What changes have taken place which have focused attention on recreation in our century? We can mention only a few.

EXPANDED LEISURE

First, and most obvious, is the possession of more leisure. Our children enter the work force later; our adults retire from labor at an earlier age, and modern technology has significantly reduced the working hours of the interim age span which mans the labor front. The recently published research from the Twentieth Century Fund predicts that by 1975 our average work week will be cut to 37 hours, with wages running up to $9,000 a year. This is a far cry from the 70-hour, $15-a-week job of 100 years ago.

Today, in America, leisure reaches all classes in ever-increasing amounts. Modern technology has provided, for the many, leisure that ancient slavery provided for the few. If you have explored Kaplan's *Leisure in America*, Alexander Reid Martin's *Philosophy of Leisure*, or Sebastian de Grazia's *Of Time, Work, and Leisure*, you will realize all too well that there is some confusion about the concept of the word leisure. We range in definitions all the way from the simplest idea that "leisure is unobligated time, time away from work and the needs of personal maintenance," to the concept that leisure is something aesthetically, morally, and spiritually valuable with no relation whatsoever to a time concept. If you will allow me to be decisive, I shall choose to describe leisure as the former—unobligated time in which one may do as he chooses.

Never before have the people of any nation had at their disposal so much free time and such varied outlets for its use. In this leisure may lie the final test of our civilization, for leisure is a two-edged sword. It may bring opportunity for the enjoyment of art, music, and science; for development of health, strength, and satisfaction; for acquisition of inner resources which lead to contentment. Conversely, it may bring boredom, idleness, overindulgence, deterioration, or corruption.

To those of you whose lives are now tremendously busy, the suggestion that leisure might cause you problems seems ridiculous. Precious free hours—three-day weekends, five-hour days—why this is the Utopia that Sir Thomas More described four centuries ago. Most problems that confront us as individuals are ones we've tried hard to avoid; yet leisure is something we've worked to created, never realizing it would bring us anything but a joyful reward. Unfortunately, the joys of leisure are sometimes not quite what we expected. It reminds me of the young, would-be naturalist who didn't get quite what he expected. As a bug and butterfly collector, he enthusiastically sent away for a book entitled, *Advice to Young Mothers.* He was quite startled when after several weeks, he received a book on baby care.

Barring a devastating war, revolution, or economic collapse, our leisure will continue to expand. Since 1900, our national productivity has increased two-thirds in possible gains in goods and services, and one-third in leisure time. With a 40-hour week and a conservative estimate for sleeping and personal maintenance, we have more than seventy hours of leisure. When we worked longer hours, it was justifiable to regard leisure as that time in which we could relax and literally re-create ourselves to get back to the job. Leisure in this century has far outstripped its re-creative needs to which it was formerly so thoroughly devoted. We must shift gears to a new concept of the worth of leisure and of recreation in that leisure. Old ideas die hard. We have worshipped the toiler, the go-getter, the burner of midnight oil. We've glorified work and condemned idleness, so that when man no longer has an excuse for his many hours of leisure which used to be given to renew the light of the fires of work, he is guilt-ridden. Leisure brings nothing but anxiety and a feeling of uselessness. For the retired person, educated to the philosophy of the godliness of industry and the sinfulness of idleness, there comes an unbearable feeling of emptiness and depression.

NATURE OF WORK

Let's look now at the changing nature of work itself. A century ago, our nation devoted itself essentially to handicraft manufacturing methods or agriculture. A man sowed his seed and reaped his crop; he was his own boss. Another took a fine piece of leather, from it created a beautiful pair of boots, and was praised for his art. One of our greatest satisfactions in life should come from our work; work used to be the means of self-realization, fulfillment, recognition. Times have changed; for a vast body of our population, work is no longer rewarding in itself. For the factory worker and sometimes for the professional in the hierarchy of bureaucracies which now exist, in the fragmentation in the fine print in our own job descriptions, leisure must be the source for creative self-realization. Those opportunities for getting a bit of ourselves expressed must come in leisure in many instances, or not at all.

CHANGING ENVIRONMENT

The third change comes in our changing environment. In a three-generation rural household, each member of the family was needed, depending on and being depended on by others. For the pioneer, no one was concerned with worry about finding adventure—new challenges came daily in just eking an existence out of the soil, the forest, or the stream. No need to conjure up ideas for expression of aggressive desires; he was testing mental, physical, and moral fibres each day. In short, opportunities for satisfactions of basic needs to keep his physical health and his psychological integrity were made to order. These included new experience and adventure, social participation, recognition in pride of achievement, response, creative experiences, and finally the security of the even rhythm of sleeping and waking, night and day, work and leisure to return to work, etc. Time meant little; actual accomplishments meant a great deal. He engaged in a kind of elemental living in which, although work took all of his energy and most of his time, he was rewarded with soundness of sleep and no need for tranquilizers.

Today we still share the same kinds of psychological needs as did our forefathers. While we have changed little, the environment in which we live has changed considerably. The twentieth century may be easier physically, but it is far from easy mentally. In our push-button era of the sixties we have yet to find one that is conveniently marked "relax"—although I understand some colleges are now offering courses in relaxation. Not a bad idea, but wouldn't it be terrible if you wound up flunking *rest*?

GROUP LIVING

A fourth change which has a real bearing on leisure and our psychological reaction to it comes in the current trend toward group living. We are segregated, truly so, not only by race, but by faith, by residential living, by schools, by age, by profession, by almost any other factor you want to name. About the only place in which we have vertical or heterogeneous grouping is in the Armed Forces. Until a young man enters the service, he may never see himself in perspective. The suburban teen-ager without a car to play "Chicken on the Highway" in his leisure considers himself an underprivileged character and he experiences all kinds of traumatic reactions if his leisure doesn't include the wherewithal—be it in tennis courts, swimming pools, or Mustangs—to keep up with the neighborhood of Joneses in which he lives. Going to grandma's farm on Sunday is no longer his idea of getting the most out of his leisure.

INCREASED INCOME

Recent years have brought higher incomes and higher purchasing power to most of the people of America. Better health, increased vitality, and higher education have all accompanied the rise in income. When income rises above that needed for subsistence, more money is available to spend for recreation. How wisely we spend that money is a matter for thoughtful concern.

CHANGING HOME LIFE

Work and recreation in early America centered in and around the home. In a three-generation home, even grandma was needed as the housework was done or the family gathered around the spinet to sing. While the home is still the basic institution in society, many modern conditions in our pushbutton age have weakened its influence in our leisure and have changed the contribution of the aged who may still live in three-generation households.

Certainly in an age of mechanization, specialization, urbanization, standardization, and materialism, when some of the symbols we worship seem to include the dollar, horsepower, atomic power, and miles per hour, recreation will play an increasingly important role in enabling persons of any age to discover themselves, to adjust to their society, to develop as total human beings.

In a future of increased disposable time, increased disposable income, and increased disposable energy, recreation is a basic human need for physical, mental, emotional, and social health. It is, moreover, no less a need for the elderly than for all other ages. In our day, in which astronauts explore space, bulldozers erase farmlands (in one state at the rate of 250,000 acres a year), our age seems likely to go down in history not as the Atomic Age, the Jet Age, or the Space Age, but as the Age of Leisure, which it is. Education for the arts of leisure, of which recreation is a part, is the challenge of our time. If we fail to accept that challenge, we may yet be termed the Age of Anxiety. If we accept the challenge and succeed, we may yet experience the Utopia that a small boy unwittingly expressed as he wrote from camp: "Dear Daddy, I send you my love. I hope you live all your life."

THE REHABILITATIVE POINT OF VIEW IN RECREATION

The basic democratic principle of the right to "life, liberty, and the pursuit of happiness" makes mandatory an increasing awareness of our obligations to groups with special problems. The aged, the ill, and the handicapped who live in our communities constitute such a minority. Much has been written of those who have entered what one author describes as the "Mild Blue Yonder." A dear friend of mine on his 65th birthday announced that he had now entered the Metallic Age—silver in his hair, gold in his teeth, and lead in his pants. All too often the lead assumes such proportions that it makes this segment of our population all but immobile. And it is not always caused by physical disability, it builds from mental depression. For others, it provides only the ballast of experience for a rough but exciting and challenging voyage on a stormy sea. Creative, meaningful opportunities in extended leisure in later maturity for both the sick and the well may make the difference.

Along with health, housing, and financial security, increased leisure in old age has become one of the greatest challenges to our present society. It's not enough just to sustain life, just to provide shelter in your nursing home, just to minister to medical needs. The challenge of our times is not to *live*, but to *live* as *fully* as possible within our physical and mental limitations.

To have years added to our lives without adequate provision for education in zestful living in those years can spell tragedy in loneliness, boredom, and discouragement for the aged in our country, wherever they live. Our present system of compulsory retirement, without careful regard to economic need, physical ability, mental acumen, or education for leisure, carries with it a psychological impact for which few retirees are prepared. You get some of the results in your nursing homes and in your homes for the aged. How then can you use recreation for rehabilitative purposes? What values can accrue from carefully planned opportunities for those aged in your care? Why should you be concerned with recreation?

Fifty years ago, health and welfare for any age were primarily exercises in humanity. Today, they have become sciences in which humanitarianism, organizational and administrative techniques, and capacity to adapt to change are all perfectly fused. Society is now seriously reevaluating its institutions and their ability and willingness to adapt to meet changing needs, but the old, familiar patterns and attitudes tend to persist.

Let's take a look at the people and the problem—or if you prefer, the "challenge" with which we are confronted. Who are these people called "the aged"? In the first place, they are individuals as different from each other as they may be from other groups. Our first mistake is to glibly lump them together into stereotypes, such as senior citizens, borrowed timers, the aged, the Golden Agers, or what have you. They represent a 35-year chronological age span, and they obviously will not fit any one recreation pattern any more than will the 20-to-55–year age group. So let's start thinking of them as individuals, with different physical and mental capacities, different social and economic backgrounds, and different interests, but with the same basic needs as any other age group.

Get rid of the stereotype—grandma with her knitting, grandpa with his whittling, and both with their rocking chairs beside their beds. As a grandmother, I resent the prototype. We can no more relegate this generation of senior citizens to the rocking chair or the television with impunity than we can allow the teen-agers to run the street in gangs with no recreative outlets. The results will be tragic in either situation.

These are *individuals*, then, in your care. Most of them grew up with a philosophy of the sanctity of work, in a society which measured human worth and dignity in terms of gainful employment. They need help in altering value structures so that attainment of 65 years, or entering a nursing home, does not necessarily mean withdrawal from life and being tossed on the social or economic scrap heap. As one author puts it, hardening of the arteries is less prevalent than hardening of the attitudes! If the aged are to have sympathetic understanding and a feeling of self-worth, there must be a more positive attitude in society toward what satisfactions leisure can hold.

The plight of the lonely, sometimes meaningless, lives of the aged should be teaching *us* some lessons at any age. When the balance of our economy demanded that we work long hours, we could justify a philosophy that sanctified diligence and deplored idleness, that used leisure as a refueling time to re-create or re-energize us to go back to work. We must remember that in earlier times most of the satisfactions of basic needs came in those work hours. But times have changed; today in our era of automation, persons at every age must look to leisure for creative outlets, adventure, new experience, service, the participation that used to be peculiar to work. Intelligent attitudes toward the value and worth of wholesome recreation at every age must be fostered so that the idea of leisure for extended periods in later maturity will not be a frightful thought, will elicit anticipation, not dread, and that regardless of age, we will seek meaningful, satisfying activity in our leisure.

We worry about the influence of television on youth, but it seems to me that all too often in our homes we have designated old age as the age of "squat and look." I have nothing against television, but, like little liver pills, it can't do everything.

Basic human needs do not change with age. Those in your care still need recognition, response, social interrelationships, physical activity, security, new experience, and change. Whatever your program in the home, it must include change. Laboratory experiments prove that man without change deteriorates, loses perspective, in short, goes crazy. Have you ever driven along an endless, straight road with no distractions by the wayside? The monotony frequently makes you withdraw as a driver; you get bored; you may go to sleep. Transfer this analogy to a life without change. If those in your care cannot change their setting, then they must have access to choices within that setting.

Recreation has been recognized as an essential ingredient in the formula for abundant living. It has also been recognized as an important adjunct to medicine. If your home is governed by prescriptions from physicians, then you work within those prescriptions—but you work with imagination and enthusiasm to provide for the elderly in their prolonged hours of leisure a gamut of recreation offerings which are physically and psychologically enriching.

The old idea of a rest cure has long since been shelved. Meaningful activity as a therapeutic tool has taken its place. In illness, a patient is more receptive to treatment if he has been happily occupied. For the healthy aged, recreation can relieve the boredom and loneliness which sometimes culminate in illness. Within his limitations, each aged person must make himself useful and wanted in his own eyes to keep his psychological integrity. Within his limitations, he must find leisure pursuits which will keep him physically active and mentally alert to prevent stagnation. The man who refuses to dress himself may expend all kinds of energy throwing a stick for the dog to chase, or playing horseshoes in the yard.

Recreation, in other words, is therapeutic in three distinct ways: first, wholesome, satisfying recreation may help keep the aged person on an even keel, physically and mentally, in this frightening, complex tempo of life in which we live; second, it can be regarded as therapy to help him on the road back to health after he has experienced illness; and third, it can be a significant factor in after-care in the home or in the community.

Recreation in any of the three settings should give opportunity to learn new interests, to improve morale, and to counteract the influences which institutionalized the patients. It should be more exciting than the symptoms of his ailment. It should provide creative outlets, personal development, social interrelationships, links to the world outside the institution, physical exercise, chances for individual pursuit of learning, aesthetic and cultural programs, and a chance for service to others. We will be looking at specific programs in another section of this chapter. I know facilities are somewhat limited; I know you are often shorthanded, but your imaginative efforts will pay off one hundred-fold. When you are tempted to relegate your patients to the rocking chair, remember that, at any age, sitting broadens you in only one area.

May I say, and with no malice, that if you do not expand your leisure opportunities for patients from humanitarian impulses, you will be forced into such expansion in the future for financial reasons by the aged who will go elsewhere because they will have been educated, we hope, to a higher plane of recreation literacy than those with whom you work today. I may be an idealist, but I cannot believe that the view from the top of the hill of life should be less beautiful and intriguing than the halfway lookout. The possible contentment in old age is expressed in this quotation, "The day is far spent and though it is allowable to lament the going of the light and the coming of the night, the twilight is sweet."

Will your home be the kind in which the aged can honestly say,

> Long long ago when Life was spring
> I thought Life was a lovely thing
> And now with snow on dale and hill
> I think so still.

PRINCIPLES OF PROGRAM PLANNING FOR THE ELDERLY

Planning is essential in almost any phase of human endeavor from which successful outcomes are expected. The builder is guided by an architect's carefully considered blueprint as he constructs the new home or school. The housewife uses time-tested recipes to make her delicious chocolate cake. The highway patrol defines a step-by-step plan to capture the fugitive. Even the law-breaker doesn't stay in business unless he has a carefully conceived *modus operandi.* Whether the end result is found in terms of people, events, buildings, or safecracking, achievement in every avenue of endeavor is firmly grounded in intelligent, creative plans toward feasible goals.

Recreation programming for the aged is no exception to this pattern. Let's take a look at a few basic principles in initiating and maintaining a recreation program for your home. I say home advisedly, for your facility should provide an environment which reflects some of the same kinds of warmth, protection, and security that the word "home" connotes. As I see it, nine major principles are involved in adequate program planning for the elderly.

1. The program should be based on individual and group needs of the people. Who are the people? As I said before, there is no prototype; physically, mentally, emotionally, they resemble or differ from each other almost as much as they differ from other age groups. Remember that they are individuals. Some are optimistic at 90, others defeated at 65. Some are bitter and resentful; others are happy and courageous. Some are serious, some jolly; some considerate, some ungrateful. Some still have physical strength and health; others are totally incapacitated; some minds are as keen as ever; some have strayed from reality. And of course there are those who range anywhere between such dichotomies.

Psychologically speaking, the aged person has a real problem because of changing status. In a youth-oriented world, in which all too often we are judged by our work output, the elderly may feel useless and unwanted. Personal circles have narrowed. The loss of old friends is keenly felt; the opportunities for making new friends are fewer. Leisure hangs heavily, and boredom encourages poor mental attitudes.

The need to be needed and to feel important again hangs like a specter. In most instances, the older person has lived in an age in which he had little opportunity to develop skills in the arts of leisure. He is apt to have been brought up by the philosophy that human dignity and worth are measured in work hours, not in free time. He may not readily accede to the idea that leisure *can* be as significant as work. He has probably dispensed with the idea of recreation as meaningless "fun and games," with no depth. A variety of imaginative approaches is needed if we are to offer old familiar activities as well as introduce new ones.

2. Inventories of interests may be helpful in getting ideas of recreation needs of patients, but the planner cannot stop there. Expressed needs are sometimes very narrow. New opportunities must be stimulated. Let's broaden the recreation horizons.

3. The program should be diverse, not only in kinds of activity but in the degree of proficiency needed for participation. We need to run the gamut from small classes, informal, drop-in, unstructured activities in two's and three's to large special events. We need to have a whole cafeteria of choices in recreation from the cultural arts to social, intellectual, and physical activities. We need to allow within each program area a chance to begin, to progress, and to master the more difficult skill outlets, whether we are talking about art, crafts, drama, dance, music, or sports.

4. Active and passive kinds of recreation should be provided with opportunities to be alone and to be in groups for enjoyment. There should be offerings which allow men to share their talents with men only, or women with women only, and those which allow the sexes to mingle. There should be activities for the bedfast, for wheelchair patients, for the ambulatory confined to the home, and for those who are physically and mentally able to engage in off-the-grounds recreation.

5. The home should be planned with enough space provision for recreation activity plus the facilities and equipment necessary for broad programming. These include a large activity room, craft room, outdoor area (active and quiet), reading room, television, record player, and movie projector.

6. Programs should be held at various times of day. Some aged are early risers; for others the evenings drag.

7. Quality leadership is necessary. There are those who would

state emphatically that only the old should lead the old; others are as enthusiastic in their belief that young faces are best to stimulate programs with the aged. Again, numbers of chronological years do not make good evaluative tools. The leader who can stimulate broad programs in recreation for the aged must know people and their needs, must know some things to do, must be able to plan and organize within flexible limits, and must be able to communicate forcefully with others to inspire them to participation. The person of any age who works with the aged, plans with the group, and possesses skills and understandings of both people and program, will find the experience with the aged a most rewarding one.

8. And, let's face it, your program depends on finances available, but I assure you that recreation is worth the money.

9. Continually evaluate your program in the light of changing needs. Be analytical, but watch out for criteria for evaluation. Lack of members shouldn't always mean dropping a program. Attempts at efficiency sometimes destroy the essence of a program.

The main thing I am asking here is that you dust off some of the things you know and try them again. One of my rural friends was asked to go to an agriculture conference recently. He refused with the statement, "No point in my going. I don't farm as well as I know how now." People are like Model T's—it sometimes take a shove or a crank to get them started. The leadership is up to you, to *be* it or to *get* it. So I hope a little of my enthusiasm for the rehabilitative values of recreation will rub off on you. Water at 100 degrees will accomplish little. At 220, it will pull freight cars. Please start operating your homes at 220 in the recreation scope. An elderly patient in a mental hospital was given a globe—his one worldly possession. One night the aide on the ward noticed that he was sleeping in a very cramped position with his arms around the globe. The aide tried to gently remove the globe, but as he did so, the old man stirred, half-wakened, and asked, "What are you doing with my world?" Can you answer his question?

VOLUNTEER LEADERS IN RECREATION FOR THE ELDERLY

Human leadership in this age of acceleration is the most essential tool in successful effort in work or in leisure. But we never have sufficient money to hire enough professionals, and, to be honest, even if we did have the money, the supply of professionals would certainly fall far short of the demand. The answer to this need is, of course, wise use of volunteers. Volunteers whom you can recruit, train, and guide in your program will not only serve you well, but they will also gain for themselves new understandings of the process of aging.

How many volunteers you need, and what skills they must have, will depend upon the variety of recreation programs you offer. But use of volunteers is not without hazard. We've all had experience with the irresponsibility of once-eager volunteers, the complaints that they are doing more than the paid workers (which may be true in some instances), the disregard for policies and procedures, or the vested interests of one kind or another. If we are going to avoid some of these hazards, sound administrative practices for use of volunteers must be established.

RESPONSIBILITY FOR VOLUNTEER SERVICES

What is everybody's business often turns out to be nobody's business. Someone on the paid staff must be charged with the responsibility of the volunteer program. He must not only work with the volunteers, suggestions for which will be dealt with later, but he must work with his colleagues to assure acceptance of the volunteer and the role which the volunteer plays. Many paid personnel resent volunteers, deny their contribution, and honestly feel that such people are threats to their jobs. The volunteer services administrator must establish the need for volunteers, communicate to staff the areas in which volunteers may give service, and establish lines of interrelationships for mutual benefit of staff and volunteers.

RECRUITMENT AND SELECTION OF VOLUNTEERS

When needs for volunteers have been established and areas of responsibility have been discussed with staff, then recruitment of able volunteers is the next step. A volunteer needs to volunteer *for something,* not given *carte blanche.* Just having bodies around will not solve your problems, but having people with a specific skill or understanding and a specific purpose to which to put that skill to use—there's the crux of the matter. The staff must be able to see the value of the volunteer. The volunteer himself must be doing something specific and satisfying enough to be able to see that he is really helping.

In recruiting volunteers, then, the first step is to see what jobs need to be done. Then recruit people who can help do those jobs. Frequently, you can get volunteers with skills that would be absolutely beyond your budget if you had to pay for them. These would include such persons as artists, musicians, public relations men, and planners. Set up policies for selection of volunteers as carefully detailed as those for professional personnel. It's extremely hard to say "no" to an enthusiastic, would-be "do-gooder," but it's twice as hard to get a misfit out of the program, once you've let him get started. Careful job specifications and job descriptions provide a firm basis for selection or rejection on an impersonal, sound basis.

ORIENTATION TO THE PROGRAM

The volunteer must be carefully and fully oriented to the philosophy under which your organization functions; the principles and procedures followed; the medical guidance under which you operate, if any; the facilities available; and the personnel structure of the organization. All too frequently volunteers make mistakes simply because they are uninformed. After orientation, opportunities for in-service training and the chance to move up the scale in terms of responsibilities taken should be considered. Few volunteers want to stay in a rut; they need specific and accomplishable goals and a clearly delineated route to more satisfying responsibilities as they progress in experience with the aged or with the program area. Intelligent assignment of volunteers to jobs they are capable of doing well will eliminate many of the frustrations of both volunteer and organization personnel.

SUPERVISION OF VOLUNTEERS

I mean supervision, not snooper-vision. The volunteer is part of your team, and as a contributing member needs the same opportunity for being observed and evaluated. Guidance on the job is mandatory to keep volunteers a healthy part of your staff.

EVALUATION AND RECOGNITION

"Thank you" for a job well done may be said in many ways. Volunteers need short-term and long-term assignments. The satisfaction of knowing that the work has been well done, the gratification of seeing his contribution help the total program may seem to be enough. Most administrators wisely give some tangible or intangible means of recognition to their volunteers. The Candy Striper at the hospital or the Pink Lady wears her uniform with pride. The youth leader proudly sports his badge. Your recognition systems and your "thank you's" may come in many ways. Armbands for volunteers give recognition and designate leadership responsibility for those who have not met the volunteer. A volunteers' *Danke schön* party at intervals helps get the idea of appreciation across. For special assignments, "Tip of the Hat" cards of wallet size have made even the self-sufficient businessman proud to display them. A New England playground system has cards which read, "Dear St. Peter, please place another star in the crown of ________________ for his service to the ____________ ____________ Recreation Department in ____________________. Sincerely, Superintendent." However you do it, say that you appreciate the time and energy spent in volunteer service.

As a final thought, please recognize that volunteers only *supplement,* they do not *replace* professional staff. Careful selection is needed, and assignments should be made by matching needs and skills. Tasks must be specific and measurable in accomplishment in a relatively short period of time. The volunteer should grow with his job with your guidance. He should be recognized frequently for his contribution. Remember that the only pay he gets is his knowledge of having been a meaningful part of your organization. As his understanding of the objectives of your organization grows, so too will his loyalty to your needs grow, as he talks to his friends in the community. When you carefully select, train, supervise, evaluate, and help your volunteer leaders to achieve a better understanding of the needs of the ill and handicapped aged, who knows, the lives you save may be theirs—or your own.

Chapter 12

Program Opportunities for the Elderly

JANET R. MacLEAN, *Dr. Recreation*

The satisfaction of self-expression through the media of arts and crafts is perhaps one of the most popular types of recreation for the aged. Adapted to physical ability, art or craft projects can serve needs of the bedfast or the mentally ill. Craft rooms for painting, pottery, sculpturing, enameling, or leather tooling enhance the social as well as the aesthetic values of this program area, but simple crafts can be introduced with no special work areas involved.

ARTS AND CRAFTS

Most aged persons have had experience in some craft since in its earlier years America was a handcraft nation. The secret of reviving their interest in old skills is to ask them to teach others and to try new crafts. The following craft ideas range from the simple to the challenging, from the inexpensive to the costly, from those which can be done by physically disabled persons to those which provide therapeutic outlets for the mentally ill.

knitting	hat designing	woodworking
weaving	whittling	copper enameling
crocheting	pottery	painting
finger painting	basketry	playing a musical instrument
beadcraft	quilting	

The making of:

candles	oatmeal box cradles	papier-mâché toys
yarn dolls	placemats	mosaic vases
mobiles	yarn balls	
puppets	linoleum prints	

Paper Flower

Materials: cleansing tissues, pipe cleaner, crayons
Tools: pinking shears
Basic Steps:

1. Place 2 pieces of cleansing tissue together.
2. With pinking shears cut ½" strip from sides of tissue as indicated in Figure 12.1.

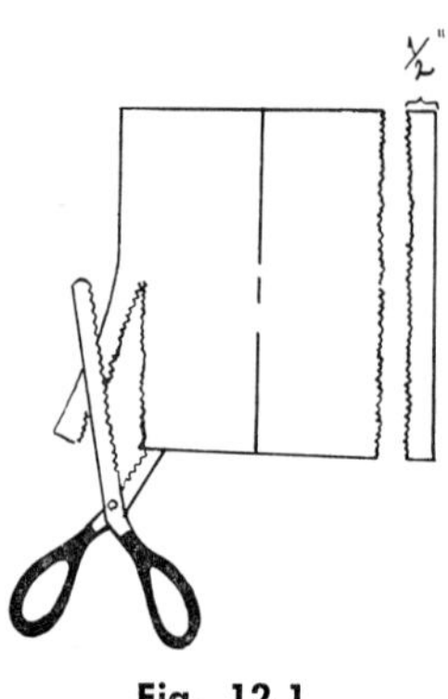

Fig. 12.1

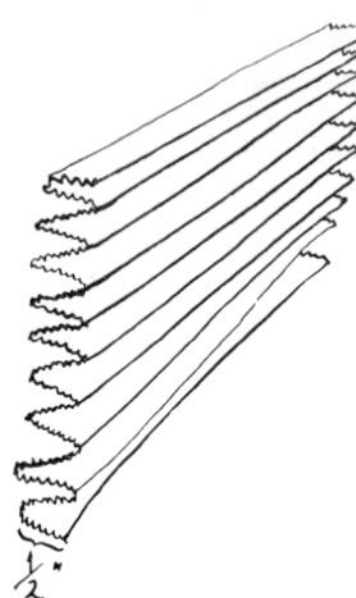

Fig. 12.2

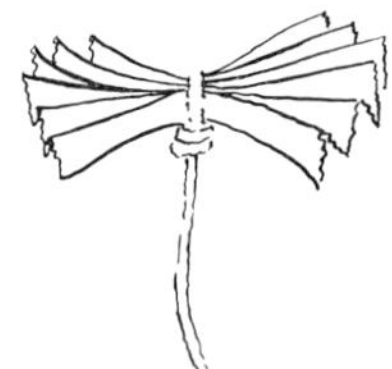

Fig. 12.3

3. Fold the tissue accordian style as shown in Figure 12.2. Each fold should be about ½" in width.
4. Wrap one end of a pipe cleaner around the folded tissue (Figure 12.3). Spread the tissue symmetrically as shown in Figure 12.4.

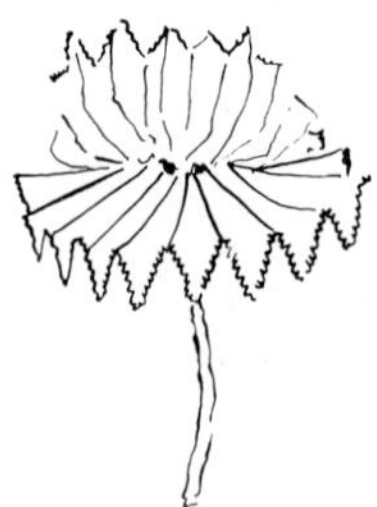

Fig. 12.4

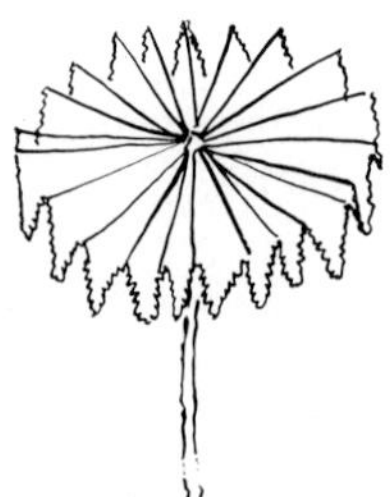

Fig. 12.5

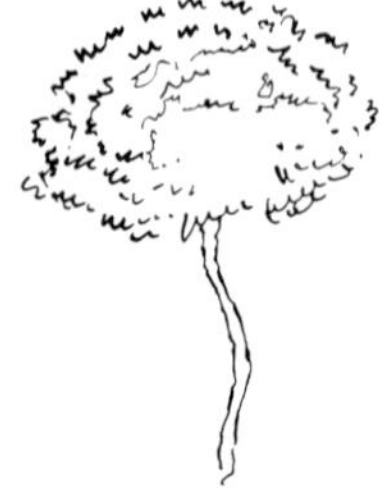

Fig. 12.6

5. Separate the top layer of tissue, 1 sheet at a time. Pull toward the center of the flower (Figure 12.5). Continue this process of separating each layer until flower is finished (Figure 12.6).

Papier Maché

Papier Mâché can take on many different shapes and forms, as illustrated in the following films, all of which may be obtained from the Audiovisual Center, The University of Iowa, Iowa City, Iowa:

How to Make Papier Mâché Animals. 22 min., sound, color. Rental: $2.75.

How to Make a Mask. 11 min., sound, color. Rental: $2.75.

How to Make a Puppet. 11 min., sound, color. Rental: $2.75.

Basic Materials for Papier Mâché: newspaper, paper toweling (or comic strips), wheat paste, water, tempera paint, alcohol, shellac, sandpaper, heavy gauge wire and string for animule, light bulb for puppet and maracas, and finely ground sawdust or modeling clay or balloon for mask.

Basic Tools: pie pan, brush, and scissors.

Basic Steps for Papier Mâché:

1. Tear newspaper and paper toweling (or comic strips) into pieces the size of silver dollars.
2. Wheat-paste mixture is made by stirring wheat paste *into* water until it forms a smooth, thick consistency.
3. Apply alternating layers of newspaper and paper toweling (or comic strips) to assure uniform covering.
4. *First layer* should be newspaper and water (except for animule). Remaining layers will be dipped in wheat paste.
5. Allow project to dry (about 1 day); sand smooth and trim; apply tempera paint and 3 coats of shellac. Clean shellac from brush with alcohol.

Animules

1. Make 3 coils of newspaper and heavy gauge wire as shown in Figure 12.7. Secure coils with string or masking tape.
2. Tie the body parts together with string or masking tape as shown in Figure 12.8. A variety of positions can be made by bending, twisting, and turning the legs, neck, body, etc.

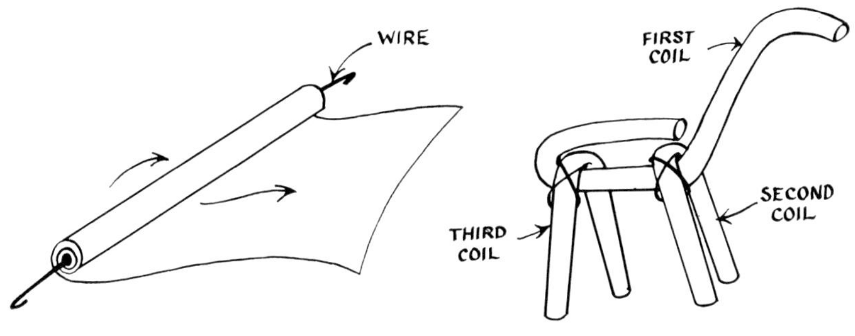

Fig. 12.7

Fig. 12.8

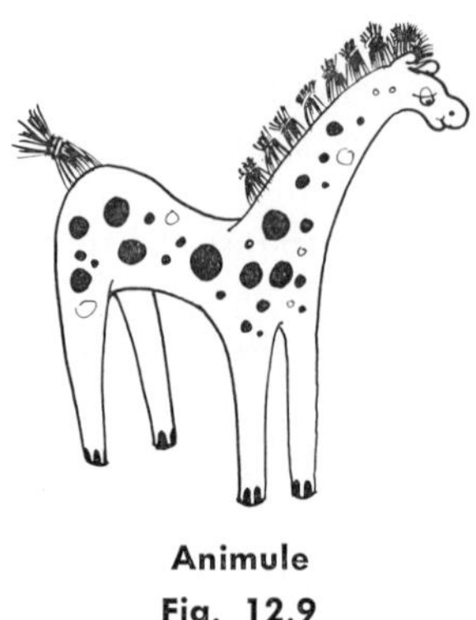

Animule
Fig. 12.9

3. To add such features as noses and ears, and to create a more realistic shape, add wadded and folded pieces of newspaper. Attach these with string or masking tape.
4. Apply 4 layers of paper as described in Basic Steps 3 and 4 (exception—first layer will be applied with wheat paste).
5. Paint and finish as indicated in Basic Step 5.

Mask

1. Mix 5 parts sawdust to 1½ parts wheat paste. Add water until mixture assumes a clay-like consistency (approximately 4 parts water). Place mixture on newspaper and shape mold. Exaggerate such features as the nose and mouth.
2. Allow mold to dry. Apply 6 layers of paper to mold as described in Basic Steps 3 and 4. When dry, remove from mold and trim edges.
3. Paint and finish as indicated in Basic Step 5.

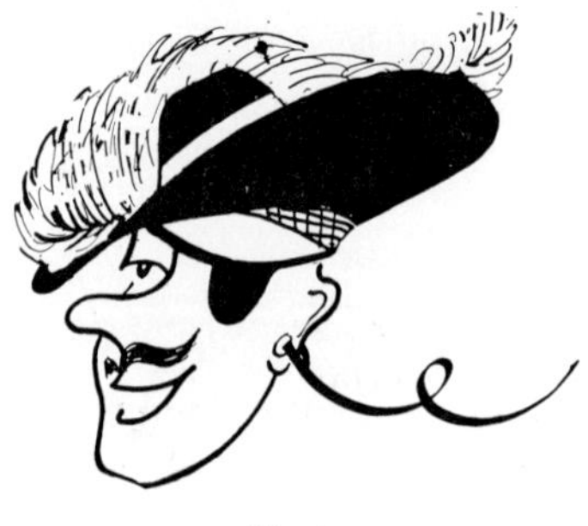

Mask
Fig. 12.10

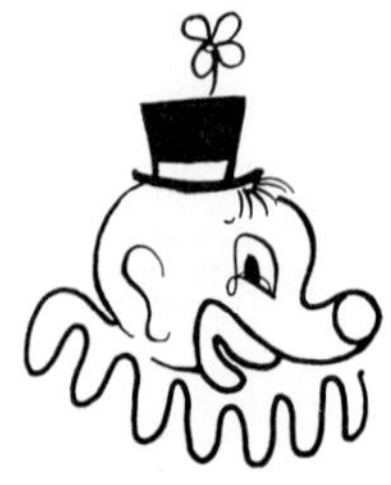

Balloon Mask
Fig. 12.11

Variation. Use modeling clay or balloon in place of sawdust–wheat-paste mixture.

Puppet

1. Cover a light bulb or a sawdust–wheat-paste mixture (follow formula for mask) with 6 layers of paper as described in Basic Steps 3 and 4 (remember to use water and newspaper for the first layer).
2. When dry, break the light bulb and remove the broken pieces from the form.
3. Paint and finish as indicated in Basic Step 5.

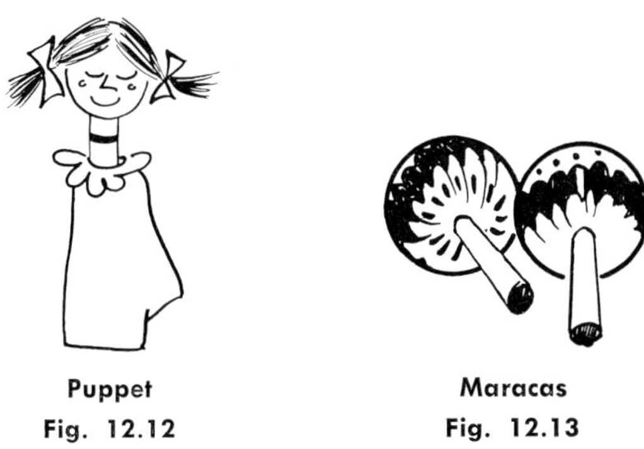

Puppet
Fig. 12.12

Maracas
Fig. 12.13

Maracas

1. Cover a light bulb with 6 layers of paper as described in Basic Steps 3 and 4. In addition, cover the bottom of the light bulb.
2. Break the light bulb so that the glass is shaking freely inside of the maraca.
3. Paint and finish as indicated in Basic Step 5.

Craft Ideas

Area	*Projects*
basketry	placemats, baskets
cork	coasters, overlays, animals
clay	modeling, tile craft
felt	pincushions, toy animals, hats
games and puzzles	bean bags, game boards, puzzles
leather	coin purses, wallets, key cases

Area (cont.)	*Projects (cont.)*
metal craft	
(a) enameling	earrings, ash trays, cuff links, pins
(b) etching	trays, bracelets
(c) tooling	name plates, pictures
(d) pounding	ash trays, dishes
musical instruments	drums, horns, whistles
paper construction	flowers, piggy bank, paper bag puppets
papier mâché	masks, maracas, puppets, animules
prints	eraser, linoleum, potato
woodcraft	chip carving, woodburning, birdhouses
yarn	wooly dog, dolls, weaving, octopus, jersey loops

Sources of Arts and Crafts Materials

Allcraft Products Co., 122 Main St., Hempstead, New York

American Art Clay Co., 4717 West 16th St., Indianapolis 24, Indiana

American Crayon Co., 1706 Hayes Ave., Sandusky, Ohio

American Handicrafts Co., 182 North Wabash Ave., Chicago 1, Illinois

American Reedcraft Corp., 417 Lafayette Ave., P. O. Box 154, Hawthorne, New Jersey

Burgess Handicraft Co., 180 North Wabash Ave., Chicago, Illinois

Cleveland Crafts Co., 4707 Euclid Ave., Cleveland 3, Ohio

Coppershop, The, 1812 East 13th St., Cleveland 14, Ohio

Dearborn Leather Co., 8625 Linwood Ave., Detroit 6, Michigan

Economy Handicrafts, Inc., 254–23 Horace Harding Blvd., Little Neck, New York

Fellowcrafters, The, 64 Stanhope St., Boston, Massachusetts

Felt Crafters, The, Plaistow, New Hampshire

Gagers, 1024 Nicollet Ave., Minneapolis 2, Minnesota

Handcrafters, The, Waupun, Wisconsin

Holiday Handicrafts, Inc., Apple Hill, Winsted, Connecticut

Horton Handicraft Company, Inc., Unionville, Connecticut

J. C. Larson Company, Inc., 820 S. Tripp Ave., Chicago 24, Illinois

Magnus Craft Materials, 108 Franklin St., New York 13, New York

Merribe Company, 2727 West Seventh St., Fort Worth 2, Texas

Metal Goods Corporation, 640 Rosedale Ave., St. Louis 12, Missouri

Peoria Arts and Crafts Supplies, 1207 West Main St., Peoria, Illinois

Puritan Plastic Corporation, Inc., 511 Lancaster St., Leominster, Mass.

Scott-Mitchell House, Inc., 611 Broadway, New York 12, New York

Tandy Leather Company, 321 East Washington, Indianapolis, Indiana

Universal Handicrafts Service, 1267 Sixth Ave., New York, New York

Selected Films on Arts and Crafts*

ABC of Puppet Making, 10 min., black and white, RS-477, $2.00 (Bailey Films, 1954)

Animules, 11 min., color, RSC-234, $3.25 (Ontario Dept. of Education and Toronto Board of Education, 1951)

Art from Scrap, 5 min., color, RSC-382, $2.25 (Crawley Films, 1955)

Block Cutting and Printing, 13 min., color, RSC-271, $3.75 (Stout Institute)

Block Printing, 12 min., black and white, RS-65, $1.75 (Universal School of Handicrafts)

Children are Creative, 11 min., color, RSC-295, $3.25 (Bailey Films)

Craftsmanship in Clay: Decoration, 11 min., color, RSC-294, $3.00 (Indiana University A. V. Center, 1951)

Craftsmanship in Clay: Glaze Application, 11 min., color, RSC-165, $3.00 (Indiana University A. V. Center, 1949)

Craftsmanship in Clay: Simple Slab Methods, 11 min., color, RSC-119, $3.00 (Indiana University A. V. Center, 1948)

Craftsmanship in Clay: Stacking and Firing, 11 min., color, RSC-189, $3.00 (Indiana University A. V. Center, 1949)

Craftsmanship in Clay: Throwing, 11 min., color, RSC-198, $3.00 (Indiana University A. V. Center, 1950)

Decorative Metal Work, 11 min., black and white, RS-19, $1.75 (Universal School of Handicrafts)

How to Make a Mask, 11 min., color, RSC-333, $3.25 (Bailey Films, 1955)

How to Make a Potato Print, 12 min., black and white, RS-396, $2.00 (Bailey Films, 1955)

How to Make a Puppet, 12 min., color, RSC-315, $3.50 (Bailey Films, 1955)

How to Make a Simple Loom and Weave, 17 min., color, RSC-447, $5.50 (Encyclopaedia Britannica Films, 1955)

Knifecraft, 11 min., black and white, NS-196, $1.75 (Boy Scouts of America, 1948)

Leatherwork, 22 min., black and white, RS-68, $3.25 (Harry A. Kapit)

Leather Work, 12 min., black and white, RS-21, $1.75 (Universal School of Handicrafts)

Let's Make Puppets, 10 min., black and white, RS-310, $2.00 (Australian Instructional Film; Library Films, Inc.)

Make a Mask, 14 min., color, RSC-238 (Crawley Films, 1951)

Pottery Making, 11 min., black and white, RS-8, $2.00 (Encyclopaedia Britannica Films, 1939)

* From *Evaluation Film Guide for Parks and Recreation,* Janet R. MacLean and Theodore R. Deppe.

Silk Screen Printing, 18 min., black and white, RS-69, $3.25 (Harry A. Kapit)

Technique of Paper Sculpture, 11 min., color, RSC-410, $3.25 (Allen Moore Production)

All the arts and crafts films listed may be rented from the Audio-Visual Center, Indiana University, Bloomington, Indiana, for the price indicated.

DANCE

For the physically able, the oldtime folk and square dances, the familiar waltzes, and the quadrilles of yesterday bring social recreation and the stimulation of movement within the restriction of physical ability. For those who are confined to wheelchairs, dance is still possible. The lively beat of the fiddler has brought wheelchair patients into activity wherever sufficient space and motivation have been provided. Dance mixers are excellent climaxing events for parties. The circle dances are good mood setters. They create a feeling of belonging for even the loneliest. Self-expression in rhythmic movement, even if only one hand is mobile, is worth the effort of the leader who creates the environment in which all handicapped persons are able to participate. Many an oldtimer would be happy to teach his clogging skill to a group in the community if opportunity were given.

MUSICAL MIXERS

Oh! Susanna. Formation: Circle of couples facing the center. Lady on partner's right.

Song:
1. I came from Alabama wid my banjo on my knee,
2. I'm g'wan to Louisiana, my true love for to see.
3. It rain'd all night de day I left,
De weather it was dry,
De sun so hot I froze to death;
Susanna, don't you cry.
4. Oh! Susanna, oh, don't you cry for me,
For I'm g'wan to Louisiana wid my banjo on my knee.
5. Oh! Susanna, oh, don't you cry for me,
6. For I'm g'wan to Louisiana wid my banjo on my knee.

Action: 1. Ladies walk four steps to center, and back. 2. Gentlemen do same. 3. Grand right and left. Partners join right hands and pass each other by, gentlemen moving counterclockwise, ladies clockwise. Continue alternating right and left hands. Counting original partner as number one, each will take seventh person he meets as a new partner. 4. Couples in skating position and promenade—counterclockwise. 5. All join hands, make a single circle facing center, and move to left. 6. With hands still joined, all go to center and back. Repeat as desired.

Shoo Fly. Formation: Single circle of couples, ladies at partner's right.

Song: 1. Shoo Fly don't bother me
2. Shoo Fly don't bother me
3. Shoo Fly don't bother me
4. For I belong to somebody
5. I do, I do, I do, and I ain't gonna tell you who
For I belong to somebody, Yes, indeed, I do.

Action: 1. Hands joined, all take four steps toward center. 2. Take four steps backward to place. 3. In again. 4. Out. 5. Repeat song if necessary. Keeping hands joined the circle is turned inside-out, by one couple lifting inside hands, and everyone else, keeping hands joined under the arch, until finally the couple making the arch turn under their own hands and the circle is still intact with everyone facing out. Repeat entire action (1) through (5). Circle becomes right side out again.

Glow Worm. Formation: Circle of couples facing counterclockwise, ladies on partner's right.

Music: *Glow Worm*
Call: 1. March, two, three, four 3. Point, two, three, four
2. Back, two, three, four 4. Turn, two, three, four

Action: 1. Partners promenade counterclockwise. 2. Partners facing each other, back away four short steps. 3. Gentleman, and lady who was in couple back of him, point to and move toward each other. 4. New partners turn or swing once around. Repeat as desired.

Lili Marlene or Susan's Gavotte. Formation: Partners standing side by side, holding inside hands. Gentleman on left.

Music: Lili Marlene

Measures:	Action:
1–2	Walk forward four steps.
3–4	Face partner, join both hands and slide to the gentleman's left, lady's right, four slide steps.
5–8	Repeat four measures in opposite direction.

9–12 Partners face, join both hands, four step-swings. Gentleman steps left, swings right foot across. Lady steps right, swings left foot across. Repeat opposite. Repeat step-swings.

13–14 Take starting position, start on outside foot. Walk three steps forward and swing free foot forward.

15–16 Repeat measures 13 and 14 in opposite direction.

17–24 Partners still hold hands and face in same direction as at start of dance. Begin with outside foot, take eight two-steps, in open position, turning toward and then away from each other. The first two-step is done facing partner, the second back to back, etc.

DRAMA

No one outgrows his need for visiting the world of make-believe. Drama in its broadest sense embodies one of the most universal of human interests. It's fun at any age to be someone else for awhile. Losing yourself in someone else's problems or joys is healthful and constructive. Drama can be introduced in the home in any of the following ways:

Play-reading clubs—even the bedfast patient can take part

Play-going clubs—for those who are mobile and free to come and go

Charades and other game activities based on dramatic expression

Puppet and marionette shows tied in with art and craft projects

Talent shows with proper staging improvised in the social hall

Skits and stunt nights

Watching television

LITERARY, MENTAL, AND LINGUISTIC ACTIVITIES

Those who like to read are never really alone. Library service is a must for recreative outlets. Talking books for the blind and ceiling projection service for the bedfast can be obtained from many libraries. Group discussion sessions on anything from philosophy to current events keep minds alert. Word puzzles, gameboards, and card games give individual and group fun. Opportunities to share creative writing experience give older people the joy of fashioning poems or prose. Letter writing may be stimulated by providing pen pals for those who have been left alone in the world. A home newspaper gives everyone a chance to catch up on community events. Storytelling for children on community playgrounds or in the local library can provide service and a rewarding feeling of being a part of the community.

MUSIC ACTIVITIES

The appeal of music is broad and music is enjoyed by every age. Tastes vary from simple, toe-tapping rhythms to classical instrumental music or choral groups. The aged love to sing; a piano or an organ is a focal point for hymn singing or the singing of popular numbers.

Music of all kinds has been cherished as a therapeutic tool to stimulate the lethargic or quiet the active. Harmonica and jew's harp bands bring back old patterns of musical expression. Rhythm band instruments can be made in the craft shop, and will furnish lively tempos as people gather for social recreation. A record player offers listening pleasures for all. The local library is a source for recordings to fit the personal tastes of all.

How To Play "Lemmi Sticks"

Music for Game

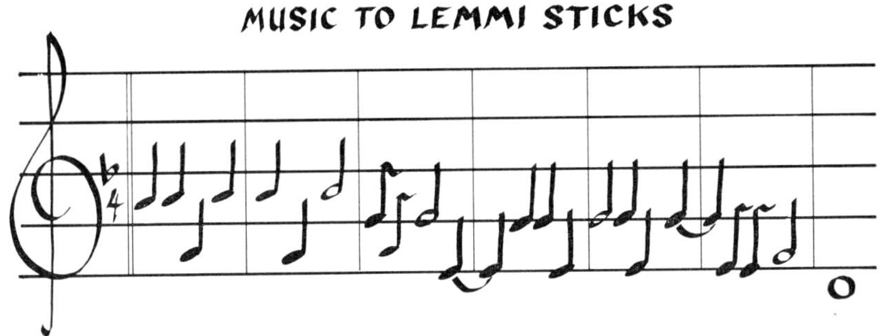

Ma-Ku Wa Kau-Te-o Wa Ku-a Tan ga
Ma-Ku Wa Kau-Te-o Wa Ku-a Tan ga

Fig. 12.14

This game is played in pairs. Each player has two round wooden sticks about 1 in. diameter and about 12–18 in. long. These may be made from dowels purchased at a hardware store or from an old broomstick. Players are seated cross-legged on floor, and face each other at about arm's length.

Five basic movements of the sticks make up this game. With these five movements any number of different patterns can be worked out. Just remember that you want *one* movement for every beat of the music. The movements are:

Fig. 1.	Clap:	hit own sticks together upright
Fig. 2.	Tap:	hit tip end of stick on floor in front; stick upright
Fig. 3.	Drum:	hit sticks on floor, tap end down
Fig. 4.	Flip:	flip sticks in air after drum, turning them once and catching other end
Fig. 5.	Toss:	throw stick to partner with an upward motion. Toss sticks gently in a vertical position

A few figures to begin with are listed below. When you've learned these let your imagination teach you the rest.

1. Tap, clap, R (right) toss, tap, clap, L (left) toss (8 times)
2. Tap, clap, R toss, L toss (8 times)
3. Drum, flip, tap, clap, R toss, L toss (4 times)
4. Tap, clap, double toss (8 times)

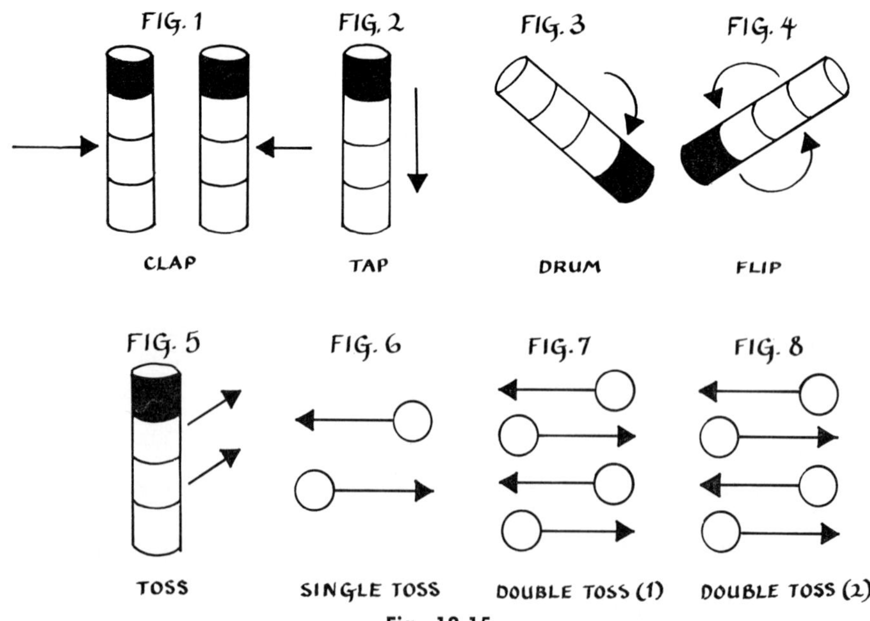

Fig. 12.15

Song Ideas

I. Starters

1. Tune: *Tipperary*

It's a good time to get acquainted
It's a good time to know
Who is sitting close beside you
So just smile and say, "hello"
Goodbye, chilly shoulder, goodbye, glassy stare
It's a good time to shout together
"We're glad that we're here."

2. Tune: *How D'ye Do*

If you're happy and you know it, clap your hands
If you're happy and you know it, clap your hands
If you're happy and you know it, then you really ought to show it,
If you're happy and you know it, clap your hands.

If you're happy and you know it, stamp your feet
Etc.
If you're happy and you know it, wiggle your nose
Etc.
If you're happy and you know it, do all three
Etc.

3. Tune: *Jimmy Crack Corn*

Clap my hands and I don't care
Clap my hands and I don't care
Clap my hands and I don't care
We're having fun today.

On third line, leader points to another person who starts a different action and song is repeated.

II. Motion Songs

1. Tune: *Down by the Station*

Down by the station early in the morning
See the little puff-a-billies all in a row
See the little driver turn the little handle
Poo-poo, choo-choo, off they go!

Down by the seashore early in the morning
See the little submarines all in a row
See the little sailor turn the little handle
Burble (finger lips to make sound of gurgling water) Off they go!

Down by the seashore early in the morning
See the little steamboats all in a row
See the little sailor turn the little handle
Whoop, whoop, whoop, (whistle sound each a pitch higher) Off they go!

Down by the airport early in the morning
See the little airplanes all in a row
See the little pilots turn the little handle
Arrrrrrrrrr (sound of planes turning) Off they go!

Down by the ranch house early in the morning
See the little horses all in a row
See the little cowboys saddle up the horses
Heheeheheheh (whinny sound) Off they go!

2. Tune: *Polly Wolly Doodle*

Directions: Sing through once with motions, then leave out section indicated and just do motion. Leave out additional section each time through. Last time, group is doing mostly motions to mental rhythm.

I push the damper in (arm straight forward),
I pull the damper out (pull arm back),
But the smoke goes up the chimney just the same (winding motion into air),
I push the damper in (repeat motions),
I pull the damper out,
But the smoke goes up the chimney just the same,
Just the same, just the same,
The smoke goes up the chimney just the same,
I push the damper in, I pull the damper out,
And the smoke goes up the chimney just the same.

3. Tune: *When You Wore a Tulip*

Are you a camel, a flip-floppy camel
Without any starch in your spine?

Do you sit at the table the best that you are able,
Or do you sit there and slump, slump, slump, slump
(slumping actions)?

Are you a camel, a flip-floppy camel, without any starch in your spine?
Well, if you are a camel, a flip-flopping camel, please go somewhere else to dine.

4. Tune: *Battle Hymn of the Republic*

It isn't any trouble just to s-m-i-l-e,
It isn't any trouble just to s-m-i-l-e,
Smile when you're in trouble, it will vanish like a bubble,
If you'll only take the trouble just to s-m-i-l-e.
(Repeat by smiling instead of singing)
It isn't any trouble just to g-r-i-n grin,
(Repeat as above)
It isn't any trouble just to l-a-u-g-h,
(Repeat as above)

III. Fun Songs With Sound

1. Tune: *When You Come to the End of a Perfect Day*

When you come to the end of a lollypop
And you sit alone with the stick,
And you think of the ones in the candy shop
Of which you would like a lick,
When you think that the taste of another one,
Would mean to an aching tongue
When this lollypop is all sucked and gone
And you long for another one.

2. Tune: *Let's All Sing Like the Birdies Sing*

Let's all sing like the goldfish sing
xxxxxxxxxx (kissing sound)
Let's all sing like the goldfish sing
xxxxxxxxxx (kissing sound)
Let's all sing like the goldfish sing
To keep the seaweed green
If there's one thing I wish bbbbbbbbbbb
It's to sing like a fish bbbbbbbbbbb
xxxxxxxxxx (kissing sound)

3. Carrousel Song

Part 1
Oom pah pah, oom pah pah, etc.
Use low voices with pitches—do, sol, sol

Part II
Omm shh shh, omm shh shh, etc.
Use as the pitch for omm

Part III
Omm tweedle tweedle, omm tweedle tweedle
Use high voices with pitches do, sol, the sol above do

Part IV
The melody part can be any song in 3/4 time such as *Bicycle Built for Two*. As the melody is sung the three rhythms are brought in separately. Continue in same tempo until the end of the melody.

4. Little Chigger (Tune: *Polly Wolly Doodle*)

Oh, there was a little chigger,
And he wasn't any bigger
Than the head of a very small pin.
But the bump that he raises just
Itches like the blazes and that's where the rub comes in.
Comes in, comes in, and that's where the rub comes in.
And the bump that he raises just itches like the blazes
And that's where the rub comes in.

IV. Rounds

1. *Scotland's Burning*

Scotland's burning, Scotland's burning,
Look out, look out!
Fire, fire, fire, fire!
Pour on water, pour on water.
(On the word fire the group may stand and shout as loud as they can.)

2. *Are You Sleeping*

Are you sleeping,
Are you sleeping,
Brother John,
Brother John?

Morning bells are ringing,
Morning bells are ringing,
Ding, ding, dong!
Ding, ding, dong!

V. Folk Songs or Campfire Songs

1. *Walking at Night*

Walking at night along the meadow way
Home from the dance beside my maiden gay.
Walking at night along the meadow way
Home from the dance beside my maiden gay. Hey!

Chorus:

Stodola, stodola, stodola pumpa,
Stodola, pumpa, stodola pumpa,
Stodola, stodola,
Stodola, pumpa, stodola pumpa, pum, pum, pum.

Nearing the woods we heard the nightingale,
Sweetly it helped me tell my begging tale.

Many the stars that brightly shone above,
But none so bright as her one word of love.

2. *Peace of the River*

Peace I ask of thee, O River, peace, peace, peace.
When I learn to live serenely cares will cease.
From the hills I gather courage,
Vision of the day to be,
Strength to lead, and faith to follow,
All are given unto me.
Peace I ask of thee, O River, peace, peace, peace.

3. *Vreneli*

"Oh Vreneli, my pretty one,
Pray tell me where's your home?"
"My home, it is in Switzerland,
'Tis made of wood and stone."

Yo ho ho, tra la la la
Yo ho ho, tra la la la
Yo ho ho, tra la la la
Yo ho ho, tra la la la
Yo ho ho

"Oh Vreneli, my pretty one,
Pray tell me, where's your heart?"
"Oh that," she said, "I gave away.
But still I feel it smart."
Yo ho ho (repeat)

"Oh Vreneli, my pretty one,
Pray tell me where's your head—"
"Oh, that I also gave away.
'Tis with my heart," she said.
Yo ho ho (repeat)

4. *Tell Me Why*

Tell me why the stars do shine,
Tell me why the ivy twines,
Tell me why the ocean's blue,
And I will tell you that's why I love you.

Because God made the stars to shine,
Because God made the ivy twine,
Because God made the ocean blue,
Because God made you, that's why I love you.

5. *Witchcraft*

If there were witchcraft, I'd make two wishes,
A winding road that beckons me to roam.

And then I'd wish for a blazing campfire
To welcome me when I'm returning home.

But in this real world there is no witchcraft,
And golden wishes do not grow on trees.

Our fondest daydreams must be the magic
To bring us back these happy memories.

Memories that linger, constant and true;
Memories we cherish, ——— (fill in name), of you.

6. *Down in the Valley*

Down in the valley, the valley so low,
Hang your head over, hear the wind blow.
Hear the wind blow, dear, hear the wind blow,
Hang your head over, hear the wind blow.

Roses love sunshine, violets love dew,
Angels in heaven know I love you.
Know I love you, dear, know I love you,
Angels in heaven, know I love you.

Build me a castle forty feet high,
So I may see her as she goes by.
As she goes by, dear, as she goes by,
So I may see her as she goes by.

7. *Old Smoky*

On top of Old Smoky, all covered with snow,
I lost my true lover by courting too slow.

For courting is pleasure and parting is grief,
But a false-hearted lover is worse than a thief.

Your grave will decay you and turn you to dust;
Not a boy in ten thousand a poor girl can trust.

OUTDOOR RECREATION

Providing outdoor recreation is a must in every nursing home or home for the aged. Grounds with trees for shade, restful contemplation or conversation, and small areas where those who love to garden can watch vegetables or flowers grow for all to admire should surround the home. Camping trips for those who are physically able; fishing and hunting for those who can leave the home on their own; are both excellent recreation pursuits. Birdfeeders provide many hours of fun and are a good woodworking project for the male residents. Audubon Clubs offer a continuing interest in life in the out-of-doors.

Weather stations and star study provide continuing areas of interest also.

For those who must be confined to their rooms for a large portion of the time, the outdoors must be brought indoors with window gardens, caged birds, herbariums, and aquariums.

PETS

This category may be somewhat unusual in a listing of recreation possibilities, but I firmly believe that a cat, a dog, or a bird is a source of relief from loneliness and boredom for the lone individual and an impetus for social interrelationships among the residents of a home. Barring physical deterrents such as allergies, pets provide hours of pleasant fun for the aged in any setting.

SOCIAL RECREATION

Social recreation—the parties, the picnics, the card games, the dances—must be carefully planned. The home where many opportunities to meet and move with others are provided has a good start toward making its residents reasonably happy. Teas, coffee hours, movies, game rooms, parties, cookouts, and interest clubs give opportunities for necessary socialization.

Here are some ideas for your next social get-together.

Mixers

Human Lotto. Prepare a sheet of paper marked into 25 squares. (16–36 if smaller or larger group.) The squares should be at least ½ in. in size. Give each person a paper as he arrives and have him introduce himself to 25 people and get each name in one of his squares. When all squares are filled, have each person in turn read one name from his sheet. As a name is read, each person checks the square on his sheet in which the name appears. The first person to have a row checked out calls "lotto."

Double Handcuff. Cut strings about 36–40 in. long. Divide the group into couples and handcuff each woman by tying an end of her string to each wrist. Then tie her partner's wrist with one end of his string, pass the other end through the loop offered by his partner, and then tie the end to his other wrist. The game is to get apart without breaking or untying the string. This looks difficult, but it is easy.

Animal Name Cards. Have some colored construction paper on hand. As guests arrive, give them a 6 in. $\times$ 6 in. piece of paper and have them tear out the figure of some animal. Place name on the animal and use as name tag. Each guest then makes a list of those present and tries to identify their name tag animals.

Musical Chairs Without Chairs. Men line up in straight line facing one way, one behind the other. Every other man places his left hand on his hip; the others place their right hands on their hips. Women hook left hands through a protruding elbow and all face counterclockwise. Have one less fellow than lady. As music starts ladies move around the circle and when music stops they must hook onto an arm—one lady to an arm.

Magazine Treasure Hunt. Divide in groups of four. Place a stock of pictorial magazines on a centrally located stand. Provide paper, paste, scissors. Try the following hunts:

1. *Find a letter.* Clip as many forms or variations of the letter (leader choose one) and mount. Time—3 minutes.
2. *Order your dinner.* Make up a complete menu and mount on paper in order of service. Time—3 minutes.
3. *Tie counter.* Clip and mount on a sheet every type and kind of tie in the magazine. Double points for ties in color.
4. *Spelling bee.* Turn to a page (leader select number) and select the most difficult word to spell you can find on the page. Clip the word and paste it on the sheet. One minute.

Chinese Puzzle. Divide people into groups of at least 14 and not over 20. Have each group form a circle holding hands firmly. A leader from each group is sent out of the room. The groups then begin to mix themselves up by moving under arms and around through their own group without breaking hands. When the group is well mixed up, the leaders come back and attempt to unwind the group as rapidly as possible. The first leader done wins. (This activity provides many face-to-face contacts.)

Eye Color. As each guest enters, he is given four cards. These are headed "blue," "gray," "green," and "brown." On them are to be listed all the people present according to the color of their eyes.

Name Acrostics. Cards and pencils are given to guests as they arrive. They are told to print their full name in capitals vertically at extreme left. Then guests move about trying to find persons whose last names begin with letters on his own card. No guest's name may be used more than once unless two people by the same name are present. (Might give 2 points for last names and 1 point for first names.) A prize may be given for the completed name based on longest name.

Circle Name Scramble. As players arrive, give each one a slip of paper and pin. Each player uses the paper as his name tag. Have players form a circle and face center. Have each one place his name tag on the floor in front of him with the name side down. The circle then moves to the left. On a signal, everyone stops, picks up the name tag in front of him and pins it on its owner. Repeat several times.

The Baby's Aunts. The "aunts" are words ending in "ant."

The youngest aunt?
The anticipating aunt?
The aunt who is never cross?
The aunt who expresses richness?
The aunt who lives in a house?
The trustworthy aunt?
The joyful aunt?
The successful aunt?
The ruling aunt?
The aunt who serves in lieu of home?
The aunt who is green, red, and black?
The aunt who carries a flag?

Personal Scavenger Hunt. The group is divided into equal teams with one runner representing each team. The leaders call for articles (pencil, shoelace, hairpin, red sock, brown belt), and if the group members have the article, they give it to their assigned runner, who races to the leader. The first runner there receives a point for his team. At the end of the hunt, the team having the most points wins.

Ocean Wave. The group sits in a circle of chairs. The "it" stands in the center and says "right" and "left." On each command, the circle moves right or left and each person sits in a new chair. The "it" moves them quickly with the object in mind to slip in and take a seat during the confusion. The person left without a chair then becomes "it."

Reverse Buzz, Clap, Whistle to 56. The players sit in a circle. The object is to count to 56 with certain limitations placed on the procedure. When the count gets to 4 or multiples of four, or a number with four in it, the participant must say "buzz" and not the number. The number 5, multiples of five, or numbers with five in them, require a clap instead of the number. The number 7, multiples of seven, or numbers with seven in them, require a whistle instead of the number. Each time there is a clap, buzz, or whistle, the line of direction of the counting is reversed. If an error is made, the whole process starts over from "one" again. It is suggested that the start be moved around the group because of the reversing. Don't worry, all will get a chance . . . the line of count won't reach 56 the first time.

No Speaka Da Language. The room is divided into two teams. A delegate from each team comes to the leader. The leader gives them an order to be bought in a foreign store. The items may be a pound of coffee, four yards of lace, a bolt of red gingham, two cows, etc. The delegate goes back to his group and pantomimes the order until someone in his group guesses what he wants. He must not speak or form letters with his mouth. When a group guesses correctly, it gets a point, and another delegate is sent forth.

Nursery Rhyme Contest. Participants are divided into two groups. The first group sings or says a nursery rhyme. As soon as they are finished, the second group must sing one. They continue alternating until one group cannot replay with a rhyme. The opposite group then wins the contest.

Rapid Fire Artistry. Each team gathers around a writing surface (desk, table, etc.) and one member is sent from each team to the leader. The leader shows the delegates a word (noun). They race back to their tables and there draw something to represent the noun they have seen. They may not write any letters and they must say nothing. The first group to guess the noun gains a point. The game is played until all members of the teams have had a chance to become delegates.

Find the Leader. "It" leaves the room. The other players select a leader who starts some motion such as clapping, making faces, stamping feet, etc. "It" is called back into the room and tries to discover who is leading the group in the frequently changing motions. When he succeeds in guessing the leader, the leader becomes "it," leaves the room, and a new leader is selected. If "it" misses three times, the leader is revealed, and the same person leaves the room while another leader is selected.

Rooster Fight. The persons are picked to represent opposite sides of the group. The director pins a small piece of colored construction paper to the middle of their backs. At the signal, the two contestants face each other, arms behind their backs, and try to see what color their opponent's paper is, without allowing their own papers to be seen. This really looks like a couple of bantam roosters in a fight. When one contestant has succeeded in correctly guessing the color, two more opponents are picked.

Adverb Expressions. Players are seated. One person is asked to leave the room. While he is gone, an adverb is chosen (sweetly, slowly, quickly). When the person returns, he may ask any individual a question. That person must answer the question honestly, but he must do it in the manner of the adverb decided upon. If the guesser asks, "What time is it?" and the adverb is "slowly," the person who answers must give the correct time in a very slow manner. Whoever gives the last answer before the person guesses the adverb correctly is "it" for the next game.

Human Tick Tack Toe. Nine seats are arranged in this formation:
X X X
X X X
X X X

Players are divided into two teams, one team on either side of the nine chairs. Each member of a team must act individually without help from any other person. First person from Team 1 sits in a chair; then the first person from Team 2 sits in a chair. Thus they alternate turns. The object of the game is to seat three in a row (diagonally, across, or up and down) for your team without letting the opposing team get three in a row. Each time a team gets three in a row it gets a point and the game starts again.

Gossip. The players sit in a circle, and the leader whispers a brief sentence to his neighbor on the right, who passes it on to the person on his right, until it has gone around the circle to the leader again. The leader then says it aloud, and gives the original sentence. Process repeated with someone else starting gossip.

Rhythm. The players are seated and number off consecutively around the room. Explain that it is not their permanent number but a number for the person sitting in that chair. A rhythm pattern is next established to a count of four: (1) slap knees once (2) clap hands together once (3) snap fingers of left hand once (4) snap fingers of right hand once. The leader is #1, and starts the rhythm. When the pattern is going strong, he says his own number (#1) on the third beat (snap of left hand), and says someone else's number on fourth beat. Whoever he calls on the fourth beat must then say his own number on the (3) third beat of the next sequence, and someone else's number on the (4) fourth beat. This continues until someone breaks rhythm or fails to call numbers in the correct order. The person missing must then go to the back of the line and take the last number. Everyone that was behind him moves up one chair and thus takes a new number, one lower. It is the idea of the game to get #1 out of his chair and try to become #1 yourself. After a miss, #1 starts the new sequence.

Shopping. A player who is the shopper walks around the circle, stops before one in the group and says, "I'm going to Denver. What can I buy?" He then counts to ten. Before he finishes counting, the player before whom he is standing must name three objects that begin with "D" (first letter of Denver), such as dishes, donuts, and dogs. If he fails, he must take the place of the shopper. Any city may be named. The things to be bought must always begin with that city's initial.

Anatomy. The leader or the person who is "it" stands before a player, points to some part of his body, and calls it by the name of some other part of his body. The player addressed must point to the part of his own body mentioned by the leader, but call it the part to which the leader pointed. For instance, the leader may say, pointing to his foot, "This is my eye." He counts quickly to ten. If the player to whom he is speaking does not point to his eye and say, "This is my foot," before ten is counted, he must become "it."

Bible Association Quiz. What person from the Bible do you associate with the items listed below:

1. The face of an angel	Stephen
2. Burning bush	Moses
3. Handwriting on the wall	Daniel
4. Locusts and wild honey	John the Baptist
5. Coat of many colors	Joseph
6. Fat king in a summer parlor	Eglon
7. A leper white as snow	Gehazi, Elisha's servant
8. Jawbone of an ass	Samson
9. Blinding light on the road to Damascus	Paul
10. Ark of gopherwood	Noah

11.	Chariot of fire	Elijah
12.	Fiery furnace	Shadrach, Meshach, Abednego
13.	Five loaves and two fishes	Jesus
14.	Ladder reaching to heaven	Jacob
15.	King's cupbearer	Nehemiah
16.	Pillar of salt	Lot's wife
17.	Walls of Jericho	Joshua
18.	Receipt of custom	Matthew
19.	Blossoming rod	Aaron
20.	Long hair in the branches of an oak tree	Absalom
21.	Sycamore tree	Zaccheus
22.	Gourd vine	Jonah
23.	Firebrands to foxes' tails	Samson
24.	Trumpets and pitchers	Gideon
25.	Five smooth stones and a sling	David

Social Recreation Activities Pattern

Here is an outline for planning social get-togethers.

Theme

Crowd

Place

Time

Plan in Detail

Invitations
Decorations
Refreshments

PROGRAM

1. Activities for First Comers
2. Mixers
3. Social Activities (Quiet and Active)
4. Refreshments
5. Climax
6. Finance

Pencil Golf

To play the game a player takes his pencil and puts it down on No. 1 tee. Then he shuts his eyes and moves pencil toward No. 1 hole. If he gets in one of the sand traps or goes out of bounds, it counts a stroke against him.

When he has moved the pencil as far as he thinks the hole is, he opens his eyes to get his bearings and moves again. The number of times he opens his eyes plus penalties is the score for that hole. Lowest number of strokes wins. Par for the course is 27 strokes, which is 3 per hole.

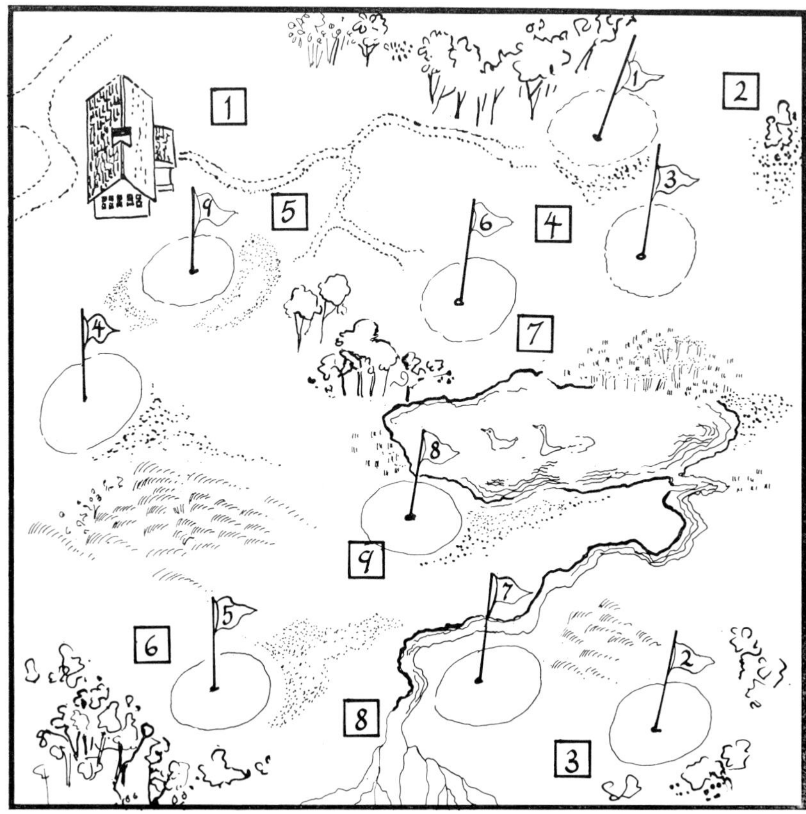

Fig. 12.16

SERVICE TO THE HOME AND TO THE COMMUNITY

The home that sets up a service outlet for its patients is doubly rewarded. Opportunities to give of whatever talent he has should be provided each person. Some are eager to cook their favorite recipes; they miss a family to eat their masterpieces. Some play instruments and can entertain others in the home; some can teach a skill in knitting, crocheting, or woodworking. Some will be physically able to go to the library, playground, or hospital for story-telling hours; others can wrap bandages or stuff envelopes for agencies in the community. As the community uses the service, people frequently become interested in the home and volunteer their talents.

SPORTS AND GAMES

The activities of oldtimers in St. Petersburg are evidence of the fact that interest in active games is still strong among the aged. Wheelchair softball and basketball are extremely popular. Croquet, horseshoes, golf putting, swimming, bowling, sailing, billiards, and shuffleboard are all popular. Tin-can golf with sunken coffee cans as holes makes for easy and inexpensive backyard courses. Bowling on the lawn is possible with plastic pins and light balls. Blacktop or concrete surfaces make possible such games as shuffleboard or four square. A tether ball or Zelball pole takes up little space but offers lively activity. Water activities, carefully supervised, are therapeutic fun. Volleyball and badminton require a minimum of equipment. The horseshoe pits are a must for the home with male patients.

SPECIAL EVENTS

Special activities add zest to the routine program of the home. Almost anything is a good enough excuse for such specials. Birthday parties, seasonal parties, special lectures, chess or checker tournaments, hobby display shows, baseball-at-the-park trips, attendance at the opera, or talent nights can highlight the daily attractions. There should be at least one "special" per week. Life loses its zest when there is nothing to which to look forward. Good leadership capitalizes on special events for any of the program areas.

TABLE GAMES

Fox and Geese

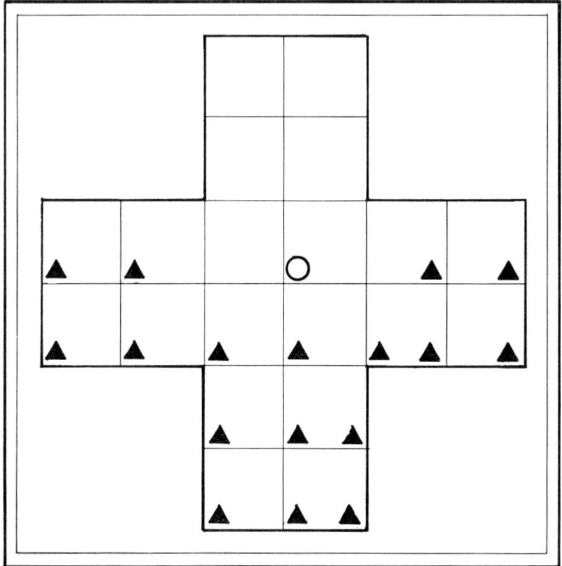

Fig. 12.17

Equipment:

A cross diagram with 33 points connected by lines as illustrated. To use pegs, drill holes. If you use marbles, countersink cups. In the old days beans and corn were often used for the 1 fox and the 17 geese.

Object:

For the geese to pen up the fox, or for the fox to capture 12 geese.

Rules:

1. Start: Begin the game with the 17 geese placed at one end of the board and the fox in the middle.

2. Moves: The fox moves first, thereafter, players alternate. Geese may move from one spot to another along the line. The fox may move in the same way, and in addition may leap over any goose to an unoccupied space beyond, or may make a series of leaps when possible. Fox is not obliged to leap when an opening appears but may move instead.

3. Capture: The fox captures and removes from the board geese that have been jumped.

4. End: The game is won by the fox if he can capture 12 geese. The geese win if they can corner the fox so he cannot move or jump. (At least 6 geese are required to pen up the fox.)

5. Notes: If the geese are played skillfully they usually win. In some cases the game is played with 15 or even 13 geese, or the geese are limited to forward moves or two foxes are entered.

Dart Baseball

The playing field is marked on a board. Permanent boards may be faced with heavy linoleum. Temporary targets may be made from beaverboard. The board should not cost more than two dollars; red and black crayons five cents each, and excellent darts may be secured from Cooperative Recreation Service, Delaware, Ohio.

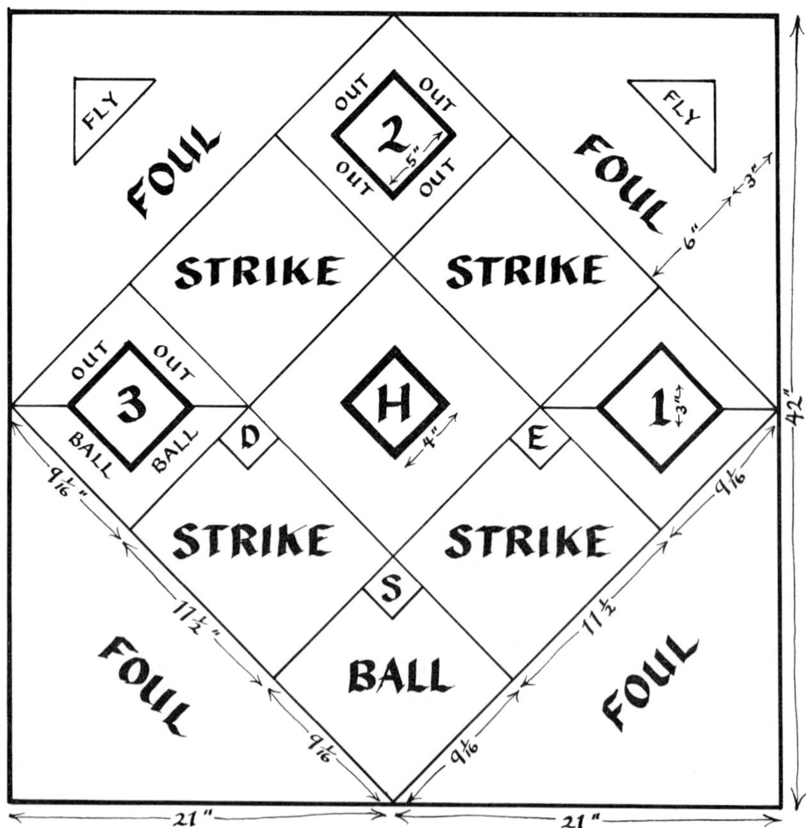

Fig. 12.18

Players follow the usual batting order of baseball. The general rules are as follows:

1. Size of board, 42 in. square. Distance from floor, 54 in.
2. Color the squares: 1, 2, 3, and H red; boundaries and lettering black.
3. The throwing distance from the board shall be 25 ft. for men, 20 ft. for women.
4. The umpire shall have complete charge of the game. It shall be his duty to call the darts, and advance darts on the board as it becomes necessary.
5. The scorekeeper shall keep score and call for "batter up."
6. If dart fails to hit board, or hits board and glances off, the batter is out. Dart hitting margin of board will be counted foul unless otherwise marked.
7. If dart hits board and falls off, or touches line, it is out.

Scoring:

8. Square (1) is a one-base hit; (2) a two-base hit; (3) a three-base hit; (H) is a home run.
9. If batter makes hit with man on base, the runner advances an equal number of bases. (Darts are moved forward.)
10. Batter hitting error (E) takes his base and any runners advance one base.
11. Batter making four balls takes his base. Runners do not advance unless forced.
12. (S) is sacrifice. Batter hitting (D) is out. Batter hitting "fly" is out.

Turtle Race

Equipment:

1. Two turtles similar to pattern (See next page)
2. Two strings 12 ft. long
3. Chair

Preparations:

1. Pass string through hole "A."
2. Fasten end of string to chair leg at about the height of the turtle from the floor.
3. Follow the same procedure with the other turtle, fastening string to the opposite leg.
4. The turtle should be near the chair legs, and inclined slightly forward.

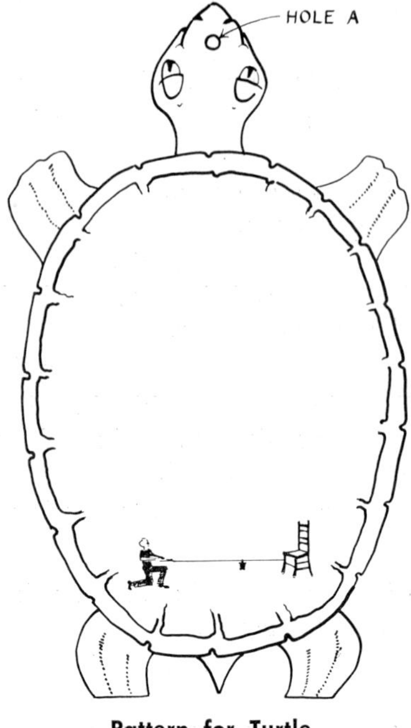

Pattern for Turtle
Fig. 12.19

Procedure:

1. The contestants stretch their strings across the room.
2. They alternately raise and lower the ends of their strings, and the turtles slide or walk on the string.
3. The contestant whose turtle reaches him first is the winner.
4. More than two turtles can race, but for best results turtles should be of similar size.

Nine Men's Morris

As shown in drawing on opposite page, playing space is 3 concentric squares with lines connecting the middle of the sides, and spots marked at the 24 intersections. Corners are not connected.

Equipment:

Each player has nine men of contrasting colors.

Object:

To capture seven of opponent's men:

1. Start with the board empty. Players take turns in placing their men one at a time to make a row of three in a line, while preventing opponents from doing likewise (not diagonally at corners).

2. If either player succeeds in forming a row of three he may remove from the board one of the opponent's men.

3. However, a row of three may not be disturbed as long as there are other men left. This rule does not prevent a player from opening his own row of three.

4. The placing continues until each man has entered his nine men on the board. This ends the first phase of the game. The second phase is "moving," the third phase "hopping."

5. After each player has placed his nine men in play, players take turns in moving a man from point to point along open lines, still attempting to make three in a row. No man may be moved twice in succession.

6. Any row of three may be opened and closed as often as desired.

7. When reduced to three men, player can hop to any point on the board.

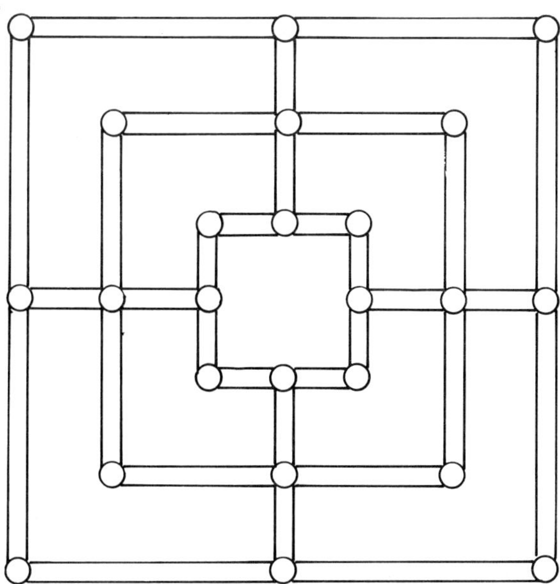

Fig. 12.20

Kicket

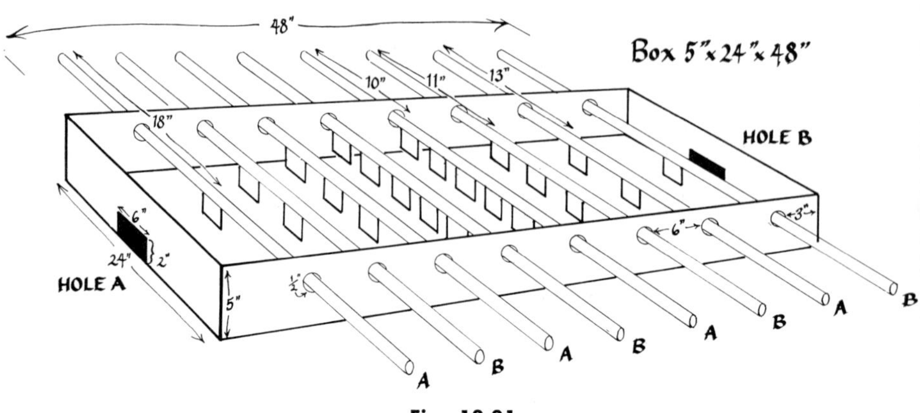

Fig. 12.21

Construction:

Box 5 in. × 24 in. × 48 in.
Each rod ¾ in. in diameter and 36 in. long.
Each paddle is 1 in. to 2 in. wide and 4 in. in length.
Box may be cut across center and hinged. Paddles of various colors may be used to help in playing.

A good way to attach the paddles to the rods is to make a saw cut in the middle of the rods, and fasten the paddles with glue and small screws. Build a shield in each corner to deflect the ball toward the goal. One-quarter-in. notches, cut down from the top edge to each side hole, permit removing the paddles for storage.

Ball:

A cork ball 1¼ in. in diameter is used (a Ping-Pong ball may be used).

Object:

Best played with four on a side. Teams stand on opposite sides, each player with one rod. To start, the ball is dropped in the middle. The goal for each team is to their left. Each goal counts 1 point with the winning score being set at 11, 15, 21, or whatever contestants decide upon.

Skittles

Playing:

The string is wound firmly around the middle part of the spindle, the end of the string pushed through the lower opening, allowing the spinner top to come through the upper hole. Balance top lightly with left forefinger. Pull vigorously back and down. A good pull will spin the top with great velocity.

If the top goes through the doors to the right or left (into the doghouses) either pin knocked down scores minus 10. If it goes out the front door and bowls over the pins in the first yard, each pin scores five points, with double score if all are bowled over. Each pin in the second yard counts 10, with double score for all. The far corners count 50, the middle room 100.

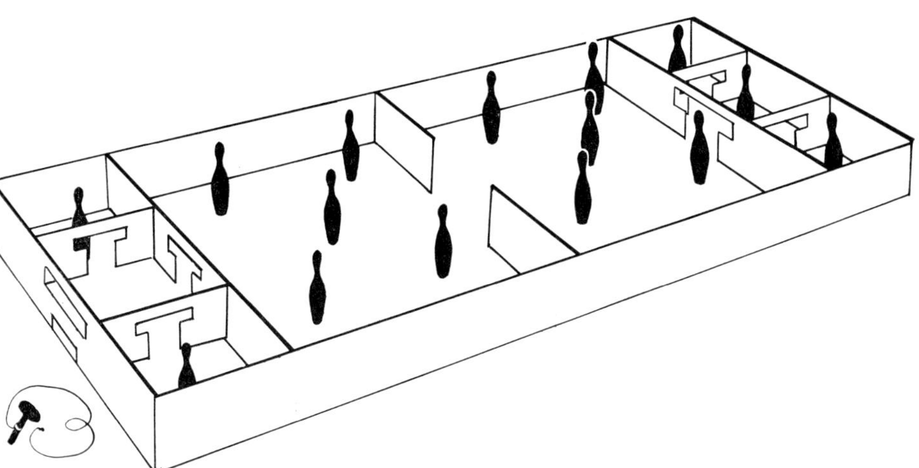

Fig. 12.22

A convenient size for skittles is 18 × 42 in., with walls about 5 in. high. The small compartments illustrated are 6 × 6 in. The center bumpers project about 5 in.

It is usually wise to rest the skittles game on a level table against a wall, and push against the box with left hand while spinning with the right. If the top has a tendency to stand still, flatten the tip slightly with sandpaper.

The fifteen tenpins are turned from a 5- or 6-in. piece of broom handle or 1-in. dowel. Those who have access to dry limbs from fruit or nut trees can turn some very beautiful and unique pins.

The spinning top is the most important part of a good game. It should be turned from a solid piece of heavy, close-grained hardwood, 6 in. long by 3 in. in diameter. When finished, the head is about 1/4 in. thick and 2 to 3 in. in diameter; the spindle about 4 in. long and 1/4 in. in diameter.

The string should be cut some 2 ft. long from chalk or fish line, with a loop in one end for the fingers.

Tether Ball

A modified game of tether ball has become very popular for indoor use. The pole has presented the greatest difficulty. The drawing at the left shows one type of pole that combines lightness with portability.

The upright is a piece of hardwood, 1 1/4 in. square and 7 to 8 ft. tall, depending on the height of the ceiling. Ash, oak, walnut, maple, or another similar wood gives best results. The corners of the upright should be rounded slightly and smoothed.

The base is constructed as illustrated. The pieces can be of the same hardwood 3/4 × 1 1/4 in. Base pieces may be 30 to 36 in. in length, the braces 20 or 24 in. long. Braces are fastened to the bases with bolts and riveted. The braces are fastened to the upright with bolts, which can be removed so that the whole base can be collapsed and carried from place to place. If necessary, the upright can be jointed in the middle to be carried in a car. A screw eye in the top of the pole takes the cord of the ball. Mark a ring around the pole halfway up.

Ball and Paddle:

For indoor use a small, sponge-rubber ball not over 2 in. in diameter is much livelier than a ball of tennis size. Smaller paddles, made of 1/4-in. fir plywood or gum plywood 6 in. wide and 14 in. long, are satisfactory.

The Game:

One player attempts to wind the ball and the string clockwise around the pole; the other tries to prevent this and wind it counterclockwise. The one who succeeds in winding the ball up, above the line around the pole, wins a point. Fouls are called (free shot to opponent) if either player strikes the pole with paddle; winds up string in paddle; or steps inside a circle drawn 30 or 36 in. around the pole.

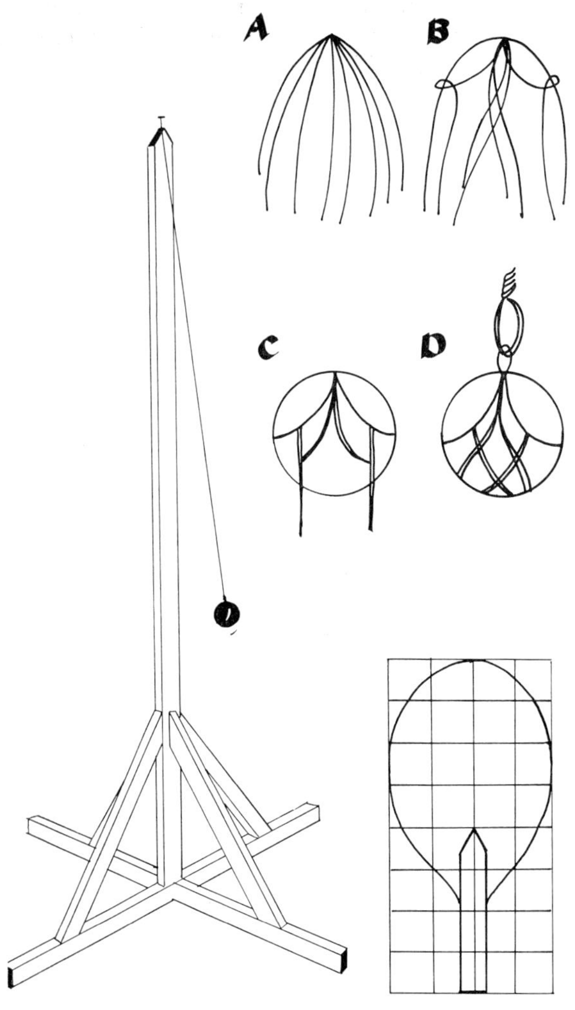

Tether Ball Equipment
Fig. 12.23

Bunum Board

Drill holes in paddle 1½ in. Drill a small hole in the top of the paddle and attach a string 24 in. to 30 in. in length. An old golf ball can be used. Toss ball in air and catch in a hole of the paddle. The numbers indicate point value of each hole. A player loses all his score if the ball is caught in the middle hole.

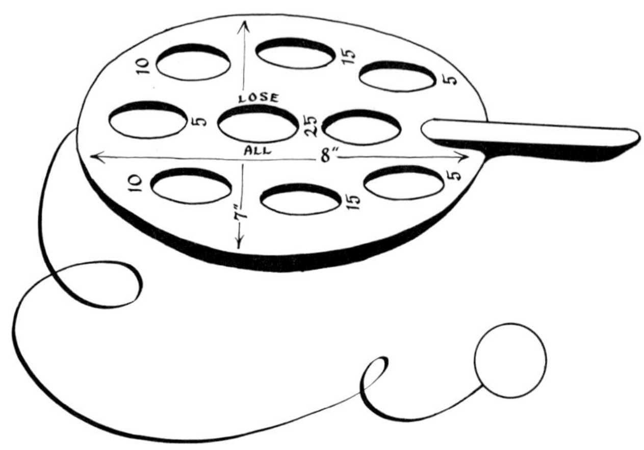

Fig. 12.24

Nine Block Puzzle

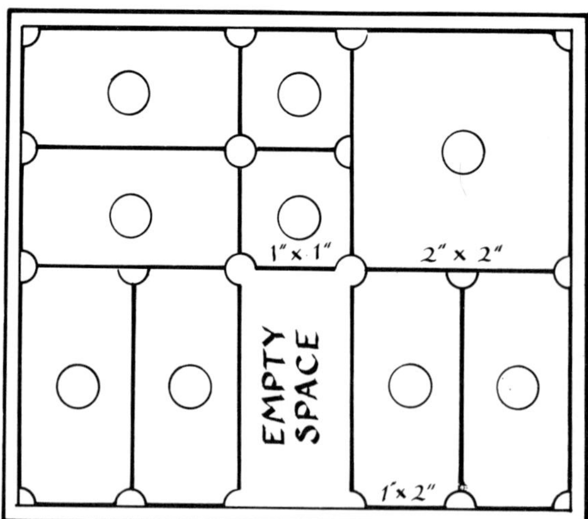

Fig. 12.25

Make base 5½ in. × 4½ in. A ¼-in. frame on base holds blocks on board. Blocks are ½ in. thick.

Object of game: To shift large block from upper right to upper left corner without lifting any block.

Part Six

EFFICIENCY IN BUSINESS MANAGEMENT

Chapter 13

Problems Involved in the Establishment of a Nursing or Retirement Home

GEORGE T. MUSTIN

A spectacular change in the health field during the past few decades has been the birth, growth, and development of nursing and retirement homes. Forty or fifty years ago, persons needing long-term care usually received it in their own homes, the county almshouse, or general hospital, depending upon their ability to meet the cost. A few establishments were operated by religious or fraternal orders, usually for the care of their own members. We now recognize them as being the forerunner of nursing and retirement homes, but their number was few and their service principally custodial. America was still largely rural.

With the mechanization of farming and the decline in farm population, families moved into towns to find work and new living arrangements. Generally, living space was less generous than on the farm, and there was a greater need for all adults to work outside the home. Consequently, no one was left to care for the elderly member of the family in need of supervisory or nursing care. Thus the need for such accommodations developed, and persons willing to undertake such care responded. The passage of the Social Security Act in the mid-1930's gave this movement greater impetus. Since that time, nursing and retirement homes have increased greatly in number and, with the passage of state laws requiring licensing and control, have advanced in quality of care.

Statistics compiled on the number of homes or the number of beds or the number of professional nurses working in those homes become obsolete very quickly, so rapidly is the picture changing. Since licensing, general staff quality has improved, and since money to build has become available, new, functional buildings are being constructed and furnished.

PRELIMINARY CONSIDERATIONS

The majority of nursing and retirement homes are still located in converted residences. Although I do not equate good care with functional buildings, long experience in the field has convinced me it is easier to give good care in a building constructed and furnished for the purpose than in a structure originally intended for other use.

Let us consider some of the factors involved in the question of converted building *versus* designed construction. First, there is the matter of patient morale. I used to hear the argument that patients preferred the converted residence because it was homelike. It was an argument put forward by owners in an attempt to stay the hand of time, and it was not really valid. One does not hear this claim made any more, since we have so many new, attractive, centrally air-conditioned and heated buildings. Patients do prefer more attractive surroundings.

There is also the matter of employee *esprit de corps*. Having operated in both the old and the new, I know what pride, zest for service, and enthusiasm can be generated by employees in a well-planned and well-furnished building. It makes them want to do more and better; it makes them proud of the new home, and employees in this mood are extremely valuable to the home.

Finally, there is the matter of the care-buying public. Because the public is not qualified to evaluate quality of care being given, it must rely on the senses of sight, touch, and smell in selecting a home. A new home, attractively decorated and furnished with a kitchen and laundry you can show, with a lounge and recreation and reception space provided, makes a strong appeal to prospective buyers and will command higher rates for the same type of service.

It is in the light of these considerations that some of the problems involved in the initiation and establishment of a nursing or retirement home project should be discussed. These include such matters as ownership and control, the place of objectives in planning, and preliminary planning for a new facility.

OWNERSHIP OBJECTIVES

Ownership may be proprietary, a partnership, a corporation operated for profit, a nonprofit institution (such as those operated by religious, fraternal, and other groups) or governmental (city or county). All have their places in the scheme of things, if a satisfactory service is to be offered. That is to say, good service is not the exclusive property of any type of ownership or control; it is policy, management, and staff which set the level and tone of service given. More comments on the implications of different types of ownership will be included later in this chapter.

Objectives in planning should make clear the principal, fundamental reason for constructing a new facility. Is the paramount purpose to give good service, or is it to make a profit? The administrator of a profit home expects to pay all expenses and have something left over for his trouble and risk. The nonprofit home is usually expected to pay its own way—to be self-sustaining. Only the governmental home should expect not to have a favorable balance of receipts over disbursements, and it should confine its clientele to low-income and destitute citizens who cannot pay cost-of-operation rates. I do not favor county or city homes competing with proprietary or voluntary homes for patients who can pay cost-of-operation or better rates, and I think they should be denied the right to do so, provided good service is available otherwise locally or nearby. So the ethics of purpose should receive utmost consideration in planning, and only those who will steadfastly place quality of service first and hold to this purpose are worthy of caring for our chronically ill citizens. It should be the aim of every administrator to encourage this purpose.

Objectives should also include a plan in which the various elements of care and service are detailed. For example, a decision must be made as to the kind of physical accommodations to be provided: single rooms with full bath, or with two-piece bath and tub or shower in hall nearby, or with connecting bath; semiprivate room, with various bath arrangements; and three or more bed wards. My personal preference is for small single rooms and semiprivate rooms, both with full bath. Naturally, the cost of such construction would be more than average, but, with long-term financing available, this additional cost could be spread over a long time. Consideration must also be given to an attractive entrance and reception room, a recreation lounge, and dining area (some of which may be separate or combined), a central court (if the design is to be in the form of a square), and walkways and gardens (if the land site is generous) for the enjoyment of guests. Floor plans of other new homes should be studied, and, if possible, visited. The entire layout should be planned for effective, efficient operation, and the rates to be charged should be fitted to the services and accommodations to be offered. Consideration should be given in planning to the guests' viewpoint, and the building should offer the utmost in safety, convenience, and attractiveness to those living within it.

PRELIMINARY PLANNING

Before a final decision is made to build or not to build, a survey of the area must be made to determine whether or not the home which is planned will have a favorable chance for successful operation.

Here are some of the factors which must be considered:

1. Population of the area to be served. Since the Department of Public Welfare has suggested three beds per thousand population, it is necessary to have this information.
2. Number of licensed beds already available.
3. Community status of present homes. If any are unsatisfactory and not patronized, then the number of their beds need not be considered.
4. Number of beds available for the chronically ill in local hospitals, if any. In some hospitals, beds are available for nursing home patients, and, if so, this must be taken into consideration.
5. Amount of welfare payments to nursing home patients. Substantial welfare payments can be a strong factor in providing a steady flow of patients, especially where supplementation is permitted to a reasonable figure.
6. What kind of pay-rate market is to be served—welfare, welfare plus private pay, medium-rate private pay, or premium-rate private pay?
7. Availability of skilled and unskilled labor, wages paid, and other factors affecting a supply of needed labor.
8. Location of the home, its proximity to the medical center, and its accessibility to labor and patient market.
9. Finally, an estimate of all costs involved: fixed costs (such as mortgage and other principal payments, taxes and insurance), and operational costs (including labor, supplies, etc.). Labor costs should take into consideration local rates for skilled and unskilled labor, based on an employee-patient ratio of 1 to 2, depending on the size and type of home (welfare, medium rate, or premium rate). From these figures, and estimating that within 12 to 15 months, a 90 per cent occupancy will be reached and then sustained, an operational cost can be estimated. Since we are on the subject of matters financial, let me urge you to give the closest attention to the absolute need for sufficient operating cash to sustain a losing operation, perhaps for the first year or so, unless you have a built-in market for patients; for example, a substantial number from an old home to be entered as soon as the new home is ready for occupancy.

Among the trends in types of living arrangements for the elderly should be mentioned:

1. home care—either with family or alone
2. ordinary boarding houses which may accept older, nonworking guests
3. boarding homes for elderly—licensed and unlicensed
4. housing for elderly with especially designed apartments, some with eating facilities, some with nursing service available
5. retirement homes, usually operated by religious groups
6. retirement hotels, wherein each guest assumes responsibility for his or her own room, and dines out or in the hotel dining room
7. city or county almshouses, or county hospitals
8. licensed homes for the aged
9. licensed nursing homes
10. nursing home wings of general hospitals
11. chronic disease hospitals
12. general hospitals

THE GOVERNING BODY

The organizational form in which a nursing center may do business can be varied and depends on the individual situation with regard to size of operation, ability of owners, financing, tax considerations, and needs of the community. Besides single ownership and owner-operation, it might be a partnership, where several persons pool their efforts and resources to operate the business. Though a partnership is a group of individuals, it is in many respects a separate legal entity, governed by the partnership agreement. It can acquire and hold property in its own name, which can be different from the names of its partners, and in those states that have adopted the Uniform Partnership Act and also most of the others, such partnership property, if bought with partnership funds and used for partnership purposes, is free from marital rights of any spouses of the partners. Under said law one partner can bind the other partner by his acts and an outsider does not have to look for any power of attorney. Each partner is fully liable for partnership debts and obligations and the death of one partner terminates the partnership, unless the partnership contract provides otherwise. Operating as a partnership has certain advantages, including the following: ease of organization (no formal requirements necessary); lack of regulations (no special statutes regulate a partnership); freedom from filing reports; can transact intrastate business as an individual; partners cannot sue each other; a partnership may incorporate at a later time. Here is an important disadvantage to operating as a partnership: all partners are liable for debts and obligations of the partnership.

A nursing home may be organized as a corporation (a separate legal entity), and, as such, be independent of its owners or the stockholders since it is created by the state by means of a charter. The corporation being a creation of the law, its powers are determined by its charter and by statutes. Its governing body is a board of directors that determines policies which are carried out by the corporate officers. A director can also be an officer of the corporation. The money for the corporation is raised by selling shares of stock to individuals who thereby become the owners of the corporation. The definite advantage of a corporation lies first, in its continuity of operation that is independent of the life of the stockholders, and second, in the limitation of the liability of the stockholder up to the amount of the stock subscribed only. It has to make certain its acts are within the powers granted by the charter, as in most states any deal or act that goes beyond such power is void.

Becoming incorporated will certainly require legal advice and assistance in obtaining a charter and the carrying out of an organizational meeting to elect officers, a board of directors, and to draw up by-laws. These by-laws should set forth: time and place of meetings of stockholders; how meetings will be called; how the stockholders' meetings will be organized; definition of a quorum; how voting shall be carried on and how elections shall be conducted; organization of the board of directors; time and place of meetings of the board; who shall be authorized to sign contracts; formation of special committees; machinery for transfer of shares of stock, keeping of stock records, etc., and provision for declaring and paying dividends.

BOARD OF DIRECTORS

Members of the board of directors are representatives of the stockholders, but not their agents, since they are not under the control of the majority of the stockholders.

The board is not the corporation title owner; it is the manager of the business, elected by the stockholders, to operate the business for the benefit of the stockholders. In the case of a nonprofit institution, the board merely represents the founding body (church, fraternal organizations, etc.) in the operation of the facility. Although these chosen persons (officers of the corporation's board of directors) operate the business, they cannot change the character of the corporation. They receive their authority to act from the articles of incorporation. In some states directors must be stockholders; this is not true in all states. Terms of office on the board may be stated in the articles of incorporation or in the by-laws. If a member resigns, the remainder may appoint someone to fill the unexpired term. Remember this about the corporation's board of directors: it is the governing body, and the business and all its employees are under its control. This control is usually exercised through a manager or administrator. The board of directors may also adopt a set of by-laws by which it will govern its actions.

Then there is that operation created by a trust or foundation, mostly in the form of a general welfare corporation, which is somewhat different from the regular business corporation. Usually it is established by a civic-minded citizen, or group of such citizens who like to have their names memorialized for future times. Such a general welfare organization is not organized for profit and has to plough back all income into its operation. It is usually governed by a board of trustees whose members serve without remuneration and are selected for their experience, knowledge, and influence in the field of operation. The actual work is done by employees under various titles and names.

Such a board of trustees is not to be confused with a board of trustees that might be attached to a highly specialized business corporation and consist of experts in the field of operation acting only in an advisory capacity. In some cases the directors of a business corporation call themselves trustees while in fact they fulfill the same functions as provided in the statute for the directors.

GETTING THE PROJECT UNDER WAY

Getting the project under way will require a number of steps taken in orderly fashion. An architect must be chosen; decisions made as to construction or conversion; site chosen (if a new building is to be constructed); the architect's plans drawn and approved; financing arranged; approval of all pertinent authorities as to site and plans obtained; and contracts let.

The architect should be chosen early so that he can be consulted about the site, planning details and questions concerning proper approval and clearance from local and state officials.

Before a site can be chosen, however, it will be necessary to decide on the size of the home—is it to be a one- or multiple-storied building? Regulations must be checked as to side and rear yards, distance set off from the street, off-street parking requirements, and availability of utilities. Possibly soil tests will need to be made. Cost is also an important consideration; the architect can be helpful here. But the location of the site is a decision for ownership and management; that is, is it to be in or close to the medical center, out from the city, or in a rural area adjacent to several communities?

If the home is seeking higher-paying patients, it should be located in or near the medical center so as to be most convenient to doctors, hospitals, families, and employees. If it is to be constructed primarily for welfare-supported patients, then a less expensive location may be sought. Cost of site, cost of construction, and long-term financing are important factors, if welfare-assisted patients are to be served so that fixed costs can be as low as may be reasonably expected. Homes catering to lower-paying patients necessarily must have lower operating costs and the place to start saving on these is in the fixed items of expense such as cost of site, building and equipment, rather than on operating costs.

A decision as to the size and type of the building will depend on the existing and anticipated market. The population of the market area, the number of satisfactory available existing beds, the type of patients to be served, the amount of financial resources available, and other factors which may influence the final decision should be considered. It should be emphasized here that this is an area where the owners must have the most competent and experienced advice available.

In selecting an architect try to obtain one who has had some experience with nursing or retirement homes, and who has an established reputation and a record of successful accomplishment. He cannot, however, be expected to make countless decisions which should be the prerogative of ownership. It would be very helpful if a number of new homes could be visited and inspected by ownership, management, and the architect and important details agreed upon in that way. The home to be studied should have about the same size and architecture as the one the sponsors plan to build, and it should be old enough to have demonstrated its practicality and success as a business.

By this time the sponsors will have long ago decided on whether to build a new facility, to convert an old one, or to add to an old one. The decision here must be purely local, depending on a number of factors, mostly economic. If the decision is not hampered by economic considerations, then by all means, new construction is usually the better choice. Adding to or converting will still leave an old building with all of the handicaps inherent in an old residential home or other nonnursing home; this is a terrific hindrance in an era when the physical appearance of the home is an important factor to the care-buying public.

Although architectural services have been mentioned as having been obtained ahead of official approval, the usual method is to keep these to a minimum, sufficient to obtain tentative approval from the authorities and from the lenders. When it can be seen that the project has their approval, plans and specifications can proceed to a finish.

Approval must be obtained from the pertinent state department, usually the State Department of Health. If financing is to be through the Federal Housing Administration (FHA), a certificate of need must be obtained from the state Hill-Burton Committee. In most states, this authority is vested in the Department of Health.

The FHA is not a lending agency, but guarantees repayment if the borrower defaults. Obtaining financing through FHA is usually more complicated than obtaining it through private sources. The FHA guarantee ranges up to 90 per cent and covers land, improvements, and heavy equipment. A licensed lender, such as a bank or savings and loan company, actually lends this money, but there is little difficulty once the project has FHA approval. Savings and loan companies have the authority to lend up to 90 per cent for twenty years, but 70 per cent loans are more common. Insurance companies, too, are good sources. Nonprofit organizations, such as churches and fraternal orders, usually raise funds by means of assessments or gifts, but they may also make use of lending agencies.

The project may require approval of the county authorities and certainly of the city authorities, if it is to be located in a town of any size. City regulations pertain primarily to zoning, construction, and parking. State regulations pertain to these factors, plus the primary purpose—its use as a health facility.

The subject of financing should cover the cost of site, temporary construction money, permanent financing of the mortgage, financing of equipment purchased or leased, and (what is very often glossed over) provision for operating cash until the project is self-sustaining. Very often, sponsors of new facilities, especially those new in this field, are too enthusiastic, too optimistic, and expect too much too soon. Many times the new facility will experience substantial financial loss for months, perhaps longer than a year, before it becomes self-sustaining. Do not make the mistake of short-term and multiple financing; keep the total monthly repayments as low as possible, and have a good cash reserve to sustain the operation until it is self-supporting.

Contracts should be let on a sealed bid basis to as many reputable general contractors as will bid. The lender will require a performance bond. Have the bids returnable on or before a certain day and hour. You may wish to let bids for the equipment and furnishings, although they are usually selected and bought.

Bids on the building should be examined and discussed by the owners and the architect, and they should satisfy themselves that the successful bidder can do a good job in the time agreed upon in the contract. When you have reached this stage successfully, let the contract and get the project under way.

SELECTION AND ORGANIZATION OF STAFF

Before employing a staff it is necessary to know the size and type of home to be operated. A large home will certainly require more employees than a small one, and a nursing home more than a retirement home. But despite all planning and the employment of the personnel deemed necessary for guest or patient load, only experience will determine the number actually required. Remember the important factors:

kind of home, number of beds, and type of patients to be served. It is important to establish personnel policies so that the employer and employee will know what is expected of each other.

Personnel policies may include a written application form filed by the prospective employee which becomes a part of the employment record if he is hired.

There should then be an interview prior to employment, a probationary period of sixty to ninety days, an orientation or on-the-job training program and a thorough grounding in company policies and detailed employee duties and responsibilities. This grounding should include a discussion of working hours, salary and salary increases, overtime, promotions, holidays, vacations, leaves of absence, excused absences, sick leave and hospitalization insurance. Other matters include uniforms, employee conduct, smoking and drinking, personal phone calls, debt collection calls and garnishment notices.

It would be well to establish a list of undesirable practices:

1. absenteeism
2. habitual tardiness
3. gambling
4. any grossly negligent careless act which results or may result in personal injury or property damage
5. sleeping on company time
6. disorderly conduct, including fighting, horseplay, or the threatening, insulting, or abusing of any person
7. unfitness to work as a result of overindulgence in drink
8. drinking on the premises
9. punching another employee's time card
10. disobedience
11. stealing
12. immoral conduct
13. soliciting or accepting gifts
14. unauthorized use or possession of narcotics

Individual situations, of course, may call for different or additional measures. The goal is to be as selective as possible since the home will, in very large measure, be the sum total of the efforts of your employees.

PERSONNEL

A retirement or nursing home will need several different types of personnel, and since the nursing home will use the same types as the retirement home (plus additional types) let us analyze what a nursing home will need in order to operate.

THE ADMINISTRATOR

The administrator is the liaison between ownership and staff, the chief employee on whom basic responsibility rests.

The administrator is responsible for the operation of the home and delegates authority thus:

1. To the director of nursing service for all matters pertaining to patient nursing and personal care. Interviewing, hiring, and discharging employees in this department should be the responsibility of the director.
2. To the kitchen supervisor for menus, buying, storing, and preparing food in an economical, efficient, and sanitary manner.
3. To the housekeeper for cleanliness of buildings and for laundry operation.
4. To the maintenance man for maintaining buildings, equipment, and grounds. This might include building alterations and the installation of new equipment.
5. To the bookkeeper for accounting and correspondence. This would include the receptionist.

In departments other than nursing, the administrator should depend upon the department head for recommendations as to the selection, hiring, and discharging of employees, but the administrator should make the final decision. All other departments should realize they are in support of nursing service and should comply with the routine requests of the nursing department, without loss of time or having to transmit orders through the administrator.

In brief, the director of nursing service is under the direction of the administrator to the extent that she will deal with him rather than directly with the board. However, if the administrator is satisfied that the director is maintaining professional nursing policies and standards, he should not intrude into the realm of actual patient care. If the administrator is absent and an emergency requires a decision, the director of nursing service is considered next in command. All other departments are under the direct supervision of the administrator.

The selection of a qualified administrator is of utmost importance. If the home has fifty or fewer beds, consideration should be given to finding a combination administrator-director of nursing service. This would require locating a licensed nurse with executive ability and nursing or retirement home administration experience. It is easier to write these words than to find such a person who is available for hire. Probably most of those who meet these specifications are already owners of a home and not interested in hiring out to a new facility. If a nurse with executive ability can be retained, some arrangement can perhaps be made for her to obtain experience in administration during the months required to construct and furnish the new home.

Let us consider what is needed in an administrator of a home with more than fifty beds. This administrator need not be a nurse or at least not necessarily so. Whether this person should be a man or woman is immaterial in my view, provided the necessary qualifications are met. However, I would be less than honest if I did not admit that, qualifications being equal, a man should be chosen to administrate rather than a woman, and I would not differ with such a choice because of the psychological factors involved. Let us suppose that our home is to be in the hundred-bed class and a lay administrator is to be selected. Our first choice would be a man, if available, who has had a record of successful administration of a large, modern installation. Administrators of this type are in decidedly short supply; so we must search for someone we can get. Let us say that an administrator with satisfactory previous experience cannot be employed. What other sources are available?

A master's degree in nursing home administration is now being offered at George Washington University. A graduate of this school would certainly be entitled to receive serious consideration. Other possibilities might be a man with a degree in business administration or a man with a degree in hospital administration.

In any case, the applicant should be married, thirty years of age or older (unless of exceptional ability), and with a clean record in his field since graduation. He should have the ability to deal with many types of people: employees, patients, patients' families, doctors, suppliers' agents, and with the general public. He should have a general knowledge of the various elements which go into nursing or retirement home operation, except medical or nursing knowledge. He should not be afraid to dirty his hands or to put his shoulder to the wheel on any occasion, if the need should arise. He should realize that he is the manager of a facility (whether proprietary or nonprofit) which must pay its way and that he is responsible for seeing that it does so. He should be able to select fundamentally sound persons for employment and to see that they receive the needed orientation to carry on their assigned job. For himself, he must not think in terms of hours or days off. For others, he must be solicitous of their welfare and advancement and consistent with his obligations to his employer. He must realize, above all, that though he is indeed the manager of a business expected to pay its way and (in the case of a proprietary home) a return to its investors, a larger obligation is owed to the people entrusted to his care; he must see that they receive the care they are entitled to before profit considerations can be taken into account.

The owners (or board) owe three important obligations to the person they select for the post of administrator:

1. To see that he receives necessary training, if he is lacking in specific knowledge.
2. To see that he receives the backing of ownership, and that no employee is allowed to bypass authority.
3. And, finally (in a facility run for profit) that he be allowed to buy into the business if this is practical and it can be arranged. An owner or part-owner has reason to have a greater interest than an employee, regardless of his importance to the business.

DIRECTOR OF NURSING SERVICES

Close behind the administrator in importance would be the director of nursing services on whom the responsibility for the major function of the home rests. Let us set down the qualities of the ideal director of nursing services:

1. graduate nurse, currently state-licensed
2. academic degree
3. age 35–55
4. executive ability
5. knowledge of, and disposition toward, geriatric nursing
6. ability to organize work force
7. ability to teach and train
8. ability to guide and lead
9. forceful but tactful personality, positive in thinking and action
10. ability to make decisions quickly
11. ability to take orders from superior
12. ability to develop and sustain excellent employee morale
13. ability to furnish satisfactory record of past employment
14. good physical and mental health
15. good appearance
16. ability to deal with people
17. ability to give professional care of highest character, without corresponding institutional atmosphere
18. well-developed sense of responsibility and loyalty
19. stable home life

With respect to the staff nurse you need not set your goals so high. The following will suffice:

1. a graduate nurse currently licensed
2. age 30–60
3. good physical and mental health
4. ability to furnish satisfactory records as to past employment
5. sense of loyalty and responsibility
6. ability to give professional care of the highest character
7. ability to direct subordinates

8. ability to deal with the public
9. ability to get along with staff and patients

If licensed practical nurses are employed, they should, except for differences in training, meet the same requirements as their graduate counterparts.

Nurses' aides work under the direction of the staff nurses. Ideally, they should have one or more years of experience on the floor of a general hospital, where very excellent training is usually received. If not, they should receive in-service training, under the direction of the director of nursing service. They should be thoroughly trained in patient care and know the value of good routines. Age limits may be flexible, if physical and mental health is good. Orderlies should be trained in the care of men patients, to assist them in all necessary care and also to be available to help lift obese patients, if needed.

The housekeeper should be able to direct housekeeping personnel in all tasks, be familiar with various cleaning agents, and be constantly vigilant, so that cleanliness may be maintained.

The food supervisor should be able to cook and to direct cooking, plan menus, purchase and store food, maintain a clean kitchen, direct preparation and serving of attractive, appetizing meals in an economical fashion.

The building superintendent or maintenance man should be handy with tools and have some knowledge of carpentry, plumbing, and electricity. He should also understand maintenance and repairs of all the equipment in use. Since grounds maintenance would also come under his jurisdiction, a basic knowledge of grass, plant, and tree care would be useful. In a business where most of the employees are women, a building superintendent who makes small adjustments and repairs promptly can be quite helpful in contributing to a smooth routine.

Every employee should be expected to have the following basic traits: honesty, integrity, industry, obedience, loyalty, and cleanliness.

Honesty means that an employee will not take anything belonging to any other person or to the home.

Integrity means a faithful performance of work, whether supervised or not, and that the employee will commit no act that is contrary to policy.

Industry means the employee will keep busy at the work assigned when on duty and that the work will be performed to the best of the employee's ability, whether supervised or not.

Obedience means the employee will obey the orders given by his or her supervisors. Orders may be given for a specific time or job, or given to be obeyed until changed. It should not be necessary to repeat orders for work which is done routinely; the original order to perform the work should be sufficient.

Loyalty means that an employee will give the home his or her best possible service, mindful that it furnishes his or her livelihood. The faithful and loyal employee will endeavor to protect and advance the interests of the home at all times, realizing that in so doing, in a measure, his or her own interests are being protected and advanced.

Cleanliness means cleanliness of person, freedom from body odor, cleanliness of face, hands, hair and nails, and neatness of uniform.

Needless to say, every employee may not measure up 100 per cent to these requirements, but it is well to set high standards and try constantly to meet them. Let me emphasize that a nursing home's greatest asset is not a building, but personnel—competent, trained, experienced, dedicated personnel, striving to aid those entrusted to their care. It is the quality of care, the level of effort, the many kindnesses shown the aged, the ill, and the infirm which distinguishes and sets apart a home of the highest calibre. Strive to make yours one of this kind.

Chapter 14

Management of Housing for the Elderly

THEODORE E. HAWKINS

After such items as the ownership plan and the methods of raising needed capital (discussed in Chapter 13) have been decided upon, the matter of rates for services must be considered.

FINANCES

Nonprofit types of facilities (churches and fraternal orders) usually compute their costs plus a small amount for contingency expenses. Many charge an admission fee plus the regular monthly rate. These rates usually are all-inclusive. However, some establish a rate covering all basic services. Personal services such as hair grooming, clothing, medical expense, recreation, etc., are considered the responsibility of the individual, relative, or agency responsible for the care.

Some have been known to arrange admission contracts in exchange for an initial gift. This sort of agreement—the life-care contract—has been ruled illegal in many states. There are conditional life-care contracts which permit the individual to elect another arrangement. Under this type of contract the facility is permitted to charge the published rate for the length of service given; all other funds must be returned to the individual. Admission fees usually are established to cover a deficit incurred in capital investment, or for capital improvement and future expansion.

Proprietary facilities, because of their very nature, must include in the rate a fair return on investment and effort. This return, above operating expenses, is usually referred to as profit.

Public housing in most instances is in the unique position of being able to obtain subsidies or grants, federal, state, or city. These funds usually are used to defray building costs. Therefore, these facilities are privileged to charge only that sum which is operating cost. Also, like most nonprofit voluntary facilities, they are tax exempt. As a result we have what is known as low-rental housing either for the elderly or for other persons less fortunate.

AVAILABILITY OF PUBLIC FUNDS

To the best of my knowledge, welfare payments can be increased only by substantiating the need. This is usually accomplished by submitting cost reports to the agency or appointed authority. It should be realized that the payee must be able to defend any expenditures he makes, since these expenditures are subject to public scrutiny and challenge. Conversely, the administrator must also be in the same position as the payee. To do this, he must maintain adequate records of operating cost. This is also a prerequisite for third-party payment. The only other possible way to be paid is for services actually being rendered. This can be accomplished by a classification system. I might add that experience has shown that this is the preferred method.

BALANCING REVENUES AND EXPENDITURES

Initially, anticipated income is indicated and an estimate of possible operating cost is set up. These figures are compared and adjusted, if possible, so that the operating budget is well within the potential income. In new facilities, however, this may not be possible for a period of six months to a year. Therefore, a cash reserve is necessary to cover the difference between the operating budget and income. Inasmuch as the majority of facilities operate on a welfare program I would like to suggest that all computations be made on welfare income.

It is recognized that 60 per cent plus of the patients being cared for are welfare recipients. If you are successful in establishing the operating budget within a welfare income, the income between the welfare rate and the private rate should be a plus on the profit side of the ledger sheet. It might be well to stop here and define privately paid care. A patient who pays in this way is one whose reimbursement to the institution provides sufficient income to allow a reasonable return or profit, after the cost of care has been met.

If one is to be successful in balancing revenues and expenditures, he or she must be continually aware of the source of income and expenditures. This is usually accomplished in the larger facilities by a monthly audit and an analysis of the balance sheet. A successful business usually shows current assets to be at least twice the value of the current liabilities. The smaller facilities can survive with a quarterly statement. However, the administrator should be aware of his income and expenses as they occur. Budgeting of expenditures is extremely important, particularly in the smaller facilities.

Depreciation is often a source of operating expense which is not generally handled as such. Therefore, when it becomes necessary to replace a capital expenditure, the funds which should have been carried in an escrow account often are not available. Good business management recognizes depreciation as an expense and treats it accordingly. Proper handling of accounts receivable is very important. Delinquent accounts have been known to kill many businesses. Establish what your financial abilities are and don't allow the receivables to go beyond it. These accounts should be reviewed weekly and proper measures taken to hold them to a minimum. It is most helpful if advance payment of a one- or two-week period can be arranged. This permits sufficient time to control any possible loss of income. The largest expenditure today is for labor.

MANAGING RECORDS AND RECORDING

Standards for good records are usually determined by the legal requirements of the respective states, and those set forth by the federal government. The latter is particularly true of financial records which are related to income taxes.

Most states require a minimum amount of information recorded pertaining to the patient. In many instances much more information would be required if you were attempting to defend yourself against a libel or malpractice suit. It might be well to discuss with the attorneys for your insurance underwriters the type of information that should be recorded in a patient's record. The least one can expect to maintain in a patient's record is:

1. the personal history sheet, containing sufficient information to complete a vital statistic certificate
2. social security death claim benefit
3. physician's history sheet
4. physician's order sheet and progress notes
5. nurses' notes
6. laboratory and diagnostic reports

A jacket or folder should be started from the time of admission and all correspondence pertaining to the patient should be kept readily available in same. An item not mentioned in this list, but one that is of equal importance, is dietary records for those patients on special diets, and written menus setting forth the food served in the general diet and the modifications used as supplements for special diets.

FINANCIAL ACCOUNTS

Accounts used by the home should be determined by the accountant, if you have one. If you are not in a position to employ an accountant on a full-time basis, one should be retained as a consultant, so that adequate records may be maintained to meet your tax needs, as well as your business operations needs. We strongly recommend that these records be taken from the "Chart of Accounts," established by the United States Public Health, Education and Welfare Service, in cooperation with the American Nursing Home Association. It is our hope that as a result of this uniform Chart of Accounts, we will be able eventually to maintain uniform accounting throughout the nursing and retirement home field.

A book listing this Chart of Accounts may be obtained through your association or from the American Nursing Home Association, at a nominal fee. It might even be well for the association to conduct several accounting seminars, so that you might become familiar with the procedures used.

INVENTORY RECORDS

Most inventory records are established at the time the business is created. However, it is never too late to take an inventory of the materials on hand. Many dollars are lost or hidden in inventory. I am sure that many administrators would be more than surprised at their homes' net worth, if this were to be established by means of a complete inventory of their respective facilities. It is usually an accumulation of small items that result in large inventories.

PRESERVATION OF RECORDS

Business records are usually maintained for a statutory period of seven years. The period relating to other records may be established by state regulation or local authority.

Most medical records are maintained for a period of ten years. Storage of these records should be handled on an annual basis, and filed in such a manner that they are readily available, particularly patients' records. Metal or wood file cabinets, because of their accessibility, provide the best type of storage. However, one can purchase storage file drawers made of heavy cardboard.

MANAGEMENT OF PUBLIC RELATIONS

Public relations, as defined by Webster, constitute "The basis of association in business or society: the kind of connection, correspondence, or feeling, either perceived or imagined, existing between two or more persons."

Public relations should be the business of *everyone* associated with the facility. The actions, deeds, and attitude of the facility, as exhibited by its employees and the management, may well be the image perceived by the community.

Any institution offering services required by the community and maintaining a high level of standards will have little difficulty in getting its fair share of the market. The cost of these services should be at least comparable to those being offered by other facilities in the community. People generally are willing to pay, but expect to get fair value in return.

There are, as every administrator knows, many selling techniques, but the best one I know anything about is what might be called the "indirect" method. I refer here to the former patient who would, if necessary, be willing to return to the nursing home. Word of mouth is recognized as an excellent source of advertising.

Securing new residents through direct contact is somewhat more difficult, as the public has little interest in what you have to offer until such times as they are involved in the need for your services.

The more you acquaint people with your facility, the more direct contact you will have. Be sure that the hospitals and the doctors know that you are part of the medical facilities program in the community and that you are in a position to serve the needs of the community—and willing to do so.

CREATING A MORE FAVORABLE PUBLIC IMAGE

From a public relations point of view, the best possible thing that the administrator can do is to function as fully as possible on the community level with all the medical and para-medical groups. What better way do you have of letting the community know that you have an interest in the well-being of the citizens of your community? The question is often asked, "Where do you find the time?" My answer is that many of you will have to make the time; others will have to delegate the more menial tasks to employees, so that they, as administrators, are free to participate in community seminars and lectures pertaining to the physical and mental health needs of elder citizens.

More attention should be given to the use of mass media in publicity and advertising. Television and radio advertising has an unlimited potential in bringing the name of a home before the community, but unless you can bring the public into your facility frequently so that they can see and actually experience some of its activities, they are likely to remain unconvinced that yours is the facility where they should place their loved one.

Nursing homes should continually operate under the open-door policy. To establish a Nursing Home Day, to carry on patients' activities in which the patient's family participates on special occasions, to have a relative or friend share a meal with the patient—these are some of the best acts of public relations one could hope to accomplish.

CITIZENS ADVISORY COMMITTEE OR BOARDS

Although this has not been a general practice in proprietary nursing homes, some of the larger facilities (75 beds or more), have adopted the Citizens Advisory Committee arrangement. I am convinced, however, that the proprietary facility should consider the feasibility of establishing a board consisting of members of the medical profession, nursing profession, social service profession, and the clergy. These are the people most involved in the care of the elderly and I am sure are in a position to give good counsel.

Most nonprofit or voluntary institutions over the years have had advisory committees or boards of trustees, which usually are the policy-making boards of the facilities. Many times these become too large and are therefore somewhat cumbersome.

WORKING WITH SPECIALIZED OUTSIDERS

When one thinks in terms of specialists, he usually has reference to a specific type of service or specialty. In the nursing home field one might wish to specialize in a specific type of nursing care, such as cardiac, cerebral vascular accident, or mild mental care. Whichever you select as a specialty, you must make every effort to learn as much as possible about the special care and treatment required in that particular field. The nursing home should be staffed and equipped to meet all the needs of that specialty. Often, in the nursing home care program, it would be better to be a master of a particular type of service, rather than to try to cater to all levels of care.

THE PHYSICIAN

In working with the physician the most successful relationship may best be accomplished when the charge nurse, or person responsible for the nursing care of the patient, discusses the needs of the patient and obtains written orders from the physician. No medication or treatment should be given without written orders. Only in case of extreme emergency should the licensed nurse attempt to administer medication or treatment without written orders.

Close observation of patients will enable the nurse to recognize any changes in the patient, which might require the services of a physician. And, whenever possible, the physician should be notified promptly so as to avoid interrupting his visiting hour schedule or late night calls. Many problems can be managed very well over the phone, if the nurse is prepared to report sufficient clinical data, such as blood pressure, pulse, respiration, temperature, or a rash, swelling, or change in patient behavior. Most physicians do not want to lose contact with their patients. However, demands made on their time and the heavy case load of acute patients is reason enough for them to overlook some of the chronic, long-term patients. Therefore, it should be the responsibility of the nursing home to keep the doctor informed as to the status of his patients. This may be done either by letter or phone, preferably by the latter. Learn to know the physician's technique and his patient approach. Whenever possible, have the patient ready to receive the physician, and have the necessary equipment for the examination available at the bedside. These practices not only conserve the physician's time, but make the examination much easier.

Adequate daily nursing notes are of great value to the physician in helping him to recognize the needs of his patients and to evaluate the patients' progress or decline.

PARA-MEDICAL PERSONNEL

First and foremost, the administrator should make every effort to know what his function should be and what relationship it may have to the patient's problem. When one has some knowledge as to what the other person's function is, it is easier to relate to others, and to understand what each is attempting to accomplish. In most instances, particularly with welfare patients, the administrator is expected to be responsible for each patient's medical and social welfare. Therefore, I believe the administrator is justified when he inquires of any person or group as to the nature of their business or the function they expect to perform for the patient. This is particularly true in cases of senility. If the administrator does not act in the best interest of the patient, who will take interest and act in the patient's behalf? I believe it is obvious that relations between any person and a group are markedly improved when both have some knowledge of the other's position and function in a given situation.

RELATIONSHIPS WITH SERVICES AND TRADES

Here, I believe, the Golden Rule is common courtesy. Should a question arise regarding service or merchandise, one should first try to find out the reasons for the objection or the lack of service. Oftentimes circumstances alter situations and a little patience and understanding contribute greatly to correcting that which has been unsatisfactory.

GOVERNMENTAL AGENCIES

To date, I feel that of all agencies, the health departments or licensing agencies of the various states have been most helpful. They have offered help in many phases of patient care and safety, as well as management. They carry on programs of continuous inspection and evaluation of facilities and care and these have resulted in the upgrading of nursing home programs. I know there are those who feel that the licensing agency is a meddlesome, unnecessary evil they would prefer to do without, but when one stops to realize the rapid growth in the nursing home program, and the number of people involved, one soon recognizes that the nursing home, like any other public facility, must meet acceptable standards and have some means of regulation.

Unfortunately, although the advancement of medicine has added longevity far beyond the expectations of our society, we have made relatively little provision for the care of our older population. Consequently, little regarding the true needs of this group is known. In fact, much that we read has been based on the living habits and needs of two generations ago. Most statistical data available is based on research done five years ago.

We are coming into an era wherein we have many more senior citizens between the ages of 80 and 85 years. The most troublesome problem of the future will probably be that of domiciliary care, with supervision. Due to the age factor, I believe the real nursing problem will be one of a short duration.

If the nursing home profession is desirous of satisfactory relationships with public agencies, it must change its philosophy and begin to talk about the needs of the patient and what it costs to fulfill these needs. The general public has little concern as to whether the nursing home is making a living or a profit. Their only true concern and obligation is the welfare of the patient. For the most part, they are not aware of today's needs—including the fact that a good standard of care cannot be provided for a cost that has been predicated on estimates of ten to twenty years ago. The greatest cost factor involved in any medical care program, including nursing care, is the labor cost, which presently ranges between 50 to 60 per cent of the total cost. If the nursing home profession has any hope of maintaining high standards of care, they must make this information available and known to the general public; as well as to the governmental agencies involved, because we have reached a point where 65 to 70 per cent of all patients in nursing homes are recipients of public assistance in one form or another, and it is the tax dollar that will determine the future of the standards of care our senior citizens will receive.

Chapter 15

Principles of Home Management

FLORENCE L. BALTZ, *R.N.*

Nursing and retirement home administrators must use sound business methods and constantly seek ways to improve their financial position. Every year more demands are made upon us to improve our facilities and offer more service so that we may fulfill our rightful role in the health care community. Therefore, it is important that we buy wisely and well.

PURCHASING POLICIES

When possible, buy from local sources but only if the price is right. Whenever local vendors offer good service at acceptable prices they merit consideration. Their attitude may help build goodwill in the community and your financial success depends on this to a great extent.

Buy from reliable suppliers. Established and reputable companies are essential to your business. Focus on a few selected suppliers. Numerous administrators report the general idea of finding a good house with which to deal and continuing to patronize this concern. Don't buy from every salesman who comes in to sell his merchandise. A dealer who gets enough business from you to make your account worthwhile will give you better attention, better service, and more consideration than one who thinks of you as a roving patron. If you deal with the same supplier long enough to get acquainted, you will be treated better. You can also order by telephone or mail each week or month and reduce the time demanded for shopping or negotiating with salesmen. Price agreements can be worked out so that a cook or nurse may order without having to argue and with the assurance that the price will be as agreed on.

Buying from a given person in the store, and ordering through a given person by telephone, can speed your work and increase your certainty of getting what you think you are getting. You have better communication with your supplier if you channel it through one person, one mind, and one pattern of thinking. The individual who knows your needs and has helped you to supply them for months past can take your order faster and fill it more accurately than another individual, even though both are equally well acquainted with the products and prices of the vendor who is supplying you.

Select suppliers on the basis of service and delivery advantages. The kind of service you get may be worth more than the difference in prices between two stores or suppliers. If one delivers and another doesn't, cost for your pickup may far outweigh your small price concession. Dependability of delivery may be even more important. Safeguards against deterioration of foods, milk, vegetables, or meats during delivery may also be worth thinking about.

Buy some things locally such as canned goods; staple foods; linens; paper goods; office supplies; medical supplies purchased in quantity; housekeeping, laundry, and maintenance supplies; equipment from wholesalers; and other articles like drugs, fresh fruits, fresh vegetables, eggs, bread, milk, small-lot medical supplies, meat, fish, and poultry. Since the size of our facilities varies, it is difficult to say which method is most satisfactory. Just because your home is small doesn't mean you cannot buy wholesale or in large quantities. (See Chapter 10 for an extensive discussion of purchasing problems.)

Cooperative buying with a group of institutions could be powerful in obtaining a fair price and high quality. This method has long been used by governmental and public groups, chains, and large hotels. Recently smaller facilities have been joining together to enjoy the benefits of pooling their purchasing power and reaping reduced prices. However, under such an arrangement you do sacrifice your individuality of selection.

Individual buying offers greatest freedom and flexibility of product selection. The shrewd purchaser knows from experience who the reputable suppliers are and when and how to get year-end discounts and special sales. Plan your menus to take advantage of seasonal foods. Many times your neighbors will offer you excess garden produce or other foods.

Contract buying is a method of cutting cost and saving time. The purchaser signs an agreement with the dealer to buy in quantity in return for low prices, fast service, and quality.

Purchase supplies on a competitive basis, making sure all are quoting on the same grade and quality. Good quality is good economy. In furniture, quality is measured primarily in terms of the product's life, sturdiness, durability, maintenance, and the like. In food we look not only for nutritive values, but for color, texture, and flavor. So many times the cost of an item is minor compared to the cost of the labor of people who are to use it. Therefore, do not invest in inferior equipment nor overlook dehydrated or ready-to-serve foods.

Test new items before purchasing your total needs. When you have given such items as incontinent pads, disposable syringes, dehydrated fruits and vegetables, or puddings, a fair trial and they prove worthy, then set up your quantity criteria.

Be courteous to sales representatives; many times they have new ideas, items, and special offers to discuss, and though you may not have need or desire to buy at that time, sooner or later you may need this product.

Listen attentively to the calling salesman. He will be a good teacher if you are a good pupil. When considering an article ask pertinent questions and whether there is a substitute that might be better at a lower price. His answers can be tested against those of two or more other firms, at least until you are satisfied you have a competent sales representative or supplier. Counseling is the main function of a salesman. If you can't trust the counsel, you can't trust the merchandise and you had better get a new vendor. Any item is only as good as the firm that stands behind it.

When buying equipment and furnishings much time and thought are required. Usually these processes begin well in advance of new construction or remodeling completion, and expert advice should be sought in the various specialized fields. Talk with representatives from several companies and get as much literature as possible on equipment; study it, then decide which would best serve your needs. The effect of equipment and furnishings upon operations and saving of labor should be fully considered.

Prudence should be exercised in purchasing, as this is definitely the place where profit or loss is determined. The person who buys food for your nursing home probably spends from 75 cents to $1 a day per person for food. If you are feeding a total of 25 patients and staff, this amounts to from $6,833 to $9,125 a year. That amount of money is worth watching, isn't it?

As pointed out previously, there are ways of quantity buying, even though in a small business. However, buying in large quantities is not always the cheapest. It is most important not to overbuy and tie up funds unnecessarily. It is wise to determine if the savings will more than make up the interest on the money tied up on the shelves. Your staple food order may account for one-third to one-half of the monthly food budget and represents a substantial investment. Prevent overbuying by making out your order as carefully as possible.

THE FOOD PLANNER

A food planner is helpful for this segment of buying. After your menus are prepared for the next month, count the number of times a given item appears on the menu, then figure the number of times it appears for the balance of the current month, total these two, determine size and number of units needed per meal, times number of meals to be served, less your stock on hand. Your answer is then the amount you need to order. Buy cans of a size to match your number of servings. This is also true of packaged items. It can be costly to have leftovers. Many times they are overlooked in the refrigerator and finally are thrown out in the garbage. Once you have calculated your order your salesman can help you decide what, if any, changes you need to make. When you substitute other foods on your list because of price, be sure the food you select fits into your carefully planned menus.

A deep freeze and a walk-in cooler are valuable aids in taking advantage of good food buys, as well as making it possible to shop on a weekly basis instead of daily. Great savings may be realized by watching weekend sales at the local markets. Don't undo hours of good work by making unwise choices now. A low price on an item is an economy only if you can use it to advantage.

Discuss and consult with your nurse, cook, housekeeper, and other personnel who will be using the new supplies, as well as the old ones, and get ideas as to quality and waste. Have them help determine the minimum and maximum requirements. This does not mean that you blindly accept their say-so. If employees feel they have had a part in making a decision they will put forth every effort to make it a success and also will be more alert and keep you posted on the pros and cons of durability, efficiency, and maintenance of specific items.

Vendors should be informed of your purchasing policies. They should know (1) they are not to call on any staff member unless they have your approval; (2) that the purchase order should be signed by one who has that assigned authority; (3) that you will designate the time you would like to have them make their calls; (4) that you would like them to invoice and bill their products. You should tell them your financial status and paying ability, and when and where to deliver their products.

It is essential to build and keep a good credit rating. To do a good job of purchasing one must be aware of needs, quality, and cost of the product, vendor's reliability, inventory limits (both financial and storage), and pricing trends. The more thoroughly you know and understand your needs and can convey this knowledge to your purveyors, the more time you will save them and yourself, an item important to both parties.

STORAGE

Storage areas will vary according to the size of the facility, location, available delivery services, type of patients served, whether supplies are disposable or reusable, the amount of inventory of linen, foods, supplies, and extra equipment you wish to have on hand.

Basically, one needs storage areas for ground and building maintenance equipment and tools, general storage for disposable and reusable supplies for nursing care, linens in use and in stock, carts, foods for daily use in the kitchen, and the monthly stock perishables, frozen, canned, and staple supplies, wheelchairs, walkers, canes, and crutches which are used daily, as well as the extras on hand, storage for soaps, detergents, disinfectants, and poisonous compounds. If patients are a short-term, convalescent type rather than long-term, less space may be required for nursing equipment. Storage is needed for garbage until such can be removed from the premises. Also, there must be storage at the nurses' station for medications, nonsterile supplies, and sterile supplies.

Storage areas must be safe and in a neat condition. It is more desirable to have several storage areas than to have only two or three larger ones; then you can match items that need to be kept in cool, warm, dry, dark, or well-ventilated rooms. Shelves, bins, and compartment sizes and shapes are determined when you decide the function of the room. The location of these rooms should be close to the area they are intended to serve; thereby lessening labor cost by having employees using less time going to and from a storeroom. If you find it necessary to place shelves higher than is comfortable for a person of average height, a sturdy stepladder must be provided.

Provide locks for all storage areas and limit keys to one or two people who are responsible to you. Even day-to-day nursing and dietary needs should be under partial security. Periodically check weights or number to see that you are receiving value as stated. A good administrator can determine quite accurately what is needed and if requests seem unreasonable, start investigating. Your loyal employees help eliminate any questionable individual.

In each storeroom post a typed list, noting what is in the area. Each shelf should be marked and, as nearly as possible, everything kept in alphabetical order, starting from the right or left. Under linen, for example, arrange, alphabetically, blankets, gowns, sheets, towels. Record supplies, admission forms, nurses' notes, physicians' orders, etc. can follow the same arrangement. This systematizing will lessen the time required for an employee to try to find something.

It is important not only to rotate foods, but to rotate other items also, including linen, paper, and rubber material. If a good rotation plan is used you will always use the oldest supplies first.

To maintain a level of supplies it is necessary to know how much is needed to do the job, how soon you can get delivery, as well as how much money you can afford to have tied up in storage, and for how long. If you have a cool, dry storage space, you can buy many staple foods monthly at real savings. Flour, sugar, cereals, canned fruits and fruit juices, canned vegetables, evaporated and dry milk, shortening, baking supplies, tea, coffee, and cocoa are all cheaper when bought by the case from a wholesale dealer than when bought in small quantities from a grocer. If you will plan menus on a four-week basis and check the supplies on hand, you can prepare a monthly order with considerable ease and accuracy.

Storage of perishables demands proper refrigeration space and sufficient room should be provided but not enough, however, to encourage too much quantity buying and resultant spoilage. Leftovers should be used within 24 hours of their first preparation.

For proper food storage it is important to maintain proper refrigerator and freezer temperatures. Refrigerator temperature should be maintained at 36 degrees F. If meat is not stored in the refrigerator 40 degrees F. is adequate. The freezer temperature should be zero or below. Thermometers should be kept in refrigeration units at all times so that the temperature can be checked daily.

Bulk ice cream should be stored at from 6 to 10 degrees F.; brick ice cream may be stored at lower temperatures. The vendor supplying ice cream usually furnishes and maintains a cabinet for ice cream storage as a part of their services. The coffee maker may be furnished and maintained by the vendor supplying coffee.

Just one word of caution, when you hear someone say you must have X number of feet for storage, it is probably less than you really need. This is especially true of new facilities. In older facilities there are many more little nooks and crannies to store things in.

PRINCIPLES AND METHODS OF CONTROL

While arrangements have been made for purchasing and storage of supplies, it is very important that the administrator establish a sound supply control program to get the greatest utilization of purchases.

An administrator has a great many duties and responsibilities; therefore it is necessary to delegate part of these to other people. Ideally, one person should be responsible for the receipt, accurate accounting, storage, and distribution of supplies. Efficient ways must be developed for obtaining requisition orders from department heads, keeping purchase records with a minimum of paper work, storing the supplies, and then distributing them to staff. All these various forms can be purchased from a record company, or you may be able to purchase a new or secondhand mimeograph machine and develop your own forms.

Requisition forms should be available to the office clerk, charge nurse, housekeeper, janitor, and cook. Then, on certain days or designated hours each day or week, these forms can be given to the person assigned, either full-time or part-time depending on the size of the facility, for the filling of these requests. The person responsible for issuing supplies must keep records showing to whom the issues are made. When the inventory gets down to the reorder point, the storeroom clerk makes out a purchase order for the administrator or purchasing agent. As the supplies are received they should be checked for accuracy to make sure that you get what you pay for. Enter these amounts on the inventory form. These forms must be kept accurately. If not, pilfering is encouraged.

Do not encourage waste by placing an overabundance of supplies at the employees' disposal. There should be specific directions on the use of supplies and equipment; these should be written out and then enforced. Accompanying every piece of equipment are directions for operation and maintenance. Copies of these should be placed in the hands of the employee using the apparatus and the maintenance man, and procedures thoroughly discussed with them.

A careful check of the needs in perishable lines is essential. To get what you think is a good buy today and have it become useless tomorrow is just a waste of time, money, and effort.

Food has a habit of disappearing after the cooks have left. It is usually blamed on the 3:00–11:00 or 11:00–7:00 shift, so the best way to eliminate this problem is to have a separate refrigerator or one compartment set aside for the P.M. and night nurses' use only and place a lock on everything else in this area.

One would like to have everybody on the honor system; however, always there are those who make it necessary to set strict rules and regulations. Keeping everything under lock and key creates a great inconvenience and slows down work. If each employee is given a key, the work can be accelerated, but then most of the control is lost. Even though you assign the key or keys to trustworthy and faithful people, it is well to spot-check periodically.

Have a definite control system for the exchange of needles, syringes, light bulbs, and similar items when replacement is needed.

You may guard against stealing by removing, as much as you can, the temptation to theft by either employees or outsiders. If you leave things unchecked, unguarded, and uncontrolled, some items will be taken away, and the percentage may be high. A check and control system, even though imperfect, establishes the possibility that it might be working at a given moment and this can be a strong deterrent to the one who would take advantage of you.

Some additional ways to prevent stealing are: keep valuables in a vault or safe; keep an inventory; let everybody know there is an inventory or record of what is on hand so that anything taken will be missed and discovered. Spot-checking at irregular intervals is also a helpful device to discourage improper actions regarding other people's property.

Dismiss staff members who are poor security risks. If food or other supplies or possessions tend to disappear, a little detective work, or perhaps even allowing someone a chance to overstep and convict himself, will bring the culprit to light. To give this type of person a second chance is likely to be unwise.

Protection must be taken against damage or destruction by some residents or guests. Stealing by residents is less common in homes for the aged than in other places, but since they have no place to hide or keep or use what they steal, there is a problem of destructiveness and damage to property of the home or of other guests by some residents. Take security precautions against the theft of drugs. Medicines or drugs that might be used for self-destruction have to be kept from those patients who may unknowingly have suicidal tendencies. Many states require a locked metal box within a locked medicine cabinet for these drugs.

Guard against intruders and prowlers. A simple precaution, such as a shade on the storeroom door will deter many prowlers. After taking all precautions you may still be faced with the embarrassment of determining who is a thief. Special care must be used in implying suspicion or accusing; however, I have found it fairly successful to begin to inquire and check without pointing a finger. The guilty one usually resigns as a result of other employees' concern with "getting to the bottom of the situation" so that they also are not under suspicion.

Remember, supply control should begin from the time goods are received, accounted for, requisitioned or stocked on the nursing unit, and charges made to the resident.

PERSONNEL MANAGEMENT

No administrator can operate a nursing home single-handedly. Well-trained, interested personnel are essential. Many factors enter into determining staff needs. Payroll is a large part of operating cost and can easily be much higher than necessary if one does not manage skillfully. What one gets in service can be much or little, depending on how one selects, motivates, supervises, and trains one's staff.

Several principles or policies affect staff size.

1. State licensing authorities set certain standards to which administrators will be required to conform.

2. It is essential to maintain a sufficient staff to render a good standard of care. This number will vary depending upon the type of patients admitted. Usually, the most difficult decision is deciding upon the actual number of nursing personnel needed. Naturally, a nursing home will not only need more staff members, but will need a greater variety than a care or retirement home. Some authorities suggest figuring on a basis of 2½ nursing hours per patient per day.

For example, 2½ hours for 20 patients equals 50 hours. Divided into 8-hour shifts, this equals 6 nurses and/or nurses' aides for each 24 hours. However, other factors enter into this method of determination. For instance, if a working recreational and craft program exists in a home, it may reduce your nursing time needs by as much as 15 minutes per day per patient.

Other authorities determine staff needs on a nurse-patient ratio; one suggested ratio being 1 nurse to 7 patients. No matter how we decide upon the number required, there must be a sufficient staff to provide a consistently high level of nursing care. When too many empty beds appear, it is logical to review our personnel to find out whether we have economized on employees to the extent that patients were neglected, or were not getting the desired level of attention.

3. Consulting services of state nursing home associations may assist in establishing staff policies. Doctors may be asked if the present staffing pattern covers the services they hope to acquire for their patients.

4. A flexibility factor is needed to meet emergencies such as illness or unexpected resignations, but one dare not retain extra employees to the extent that some do not work a sufficient number of hours. Be aware of state laws regarding employment and conform to them. The Department of Labor had never checked our nursing home for the employees' working hours during the past twelve years, but just recently there have been checks in three of our newly opened facilities which have been in operation four to six weeks. There seems to be an increasing awareness of nursing home operations and the hiring of more employees.

5. Staff according to ratio of patient income. When the payroll exceeds the danger mark it is time to take corrective measures. Payroll should not exceed 50 to 55 per cent of income. If your payroll is in excess of these percentages, perhaps the work is not organized to get the most out of your present number of employees, or perhaps you are giving more service than your rate warrants. Perhaps this rate needs to be adjusted upward.

6. Advanced hiring is necessary for planned future expansion. This may call for a temporary overstaffing in some areas in order to have trained persons ready when needed.

So far, we have been speaking chiefly in numbers. In caring for patients a great many people are required. They fall generally into the following categories:

1. The administrator, who is responsible for the emotional, spiritual, social, and physical well-being of each patient, and the coordination of all departments and employees.

2. Nurses and aides, who assist in all activities which promote the general welfare of the patient, including, but not limited to,

bedside care, recreation activities, therapy programs, dining, etc.

3. The activity director, who aids in craft and recreational programs, and coordinates all volunteer services, such as ministerial associations, church, school, and civic groups, and individual volunteer workers.

4. The physical therapy department that aids in rehabilitation of the patient by the use of physical therapy techniques and equipment.

5. Dietary employees, who see that the patients have the proper food.

6. Housekeeping employees, who keep the home immaculate.

7. Laundry and linen employees, who care for linen, and the patients' laundry.

8. The maintenance man, who keeps the mechanical equipment running, the entire facility in a good state of repair, and the grounds and buildings clean and attractive.

9. The business office personnel who keep all financial and medical records, and handle the many business details that must be included in the operation of a nursing home.

10. Volunteers, who aid the activity director in doing craft work, playing games, having parties and programs, serving refreshments to the patients, and also recruiting other volunteers. They are friendly visitors and good listeners.

One or more R.N.'s should be provided; also L.P.N.'s if they are available. If you, as administrator, are an R.N. or L.P.N., this is fine, but there should be at least one other qualified person on the staff. No one manager can be in all places at all times. Some states now are, and more states will be, requiring licensed nurse coverage "around the clock." There must always be at least one qualified person on active duty at all times. These staff needs depend upon the number of residents, and also the type of resident. A number of nurses' aides are needed to cover all three shifts and some are required for relief duty as well. On the 7:00–3:00 shift there should be 1 aide to 7 to 10 patients. The number should be adjusted according to the needs of the residents in the home at various times.

Someone must tend to the cleaning, whether she is called a maid, housekeeper, or "the cleaning lady." Your kitchen must be staffed by persons capable of preparing and serving nourishing, attractive, and appetizing meals. The number of cooks and kitchen assistants will again vary with the census, the number of special diets, the kitchen arrangement, and the types of foods used.

Laundry, if done in the building, will require the services of at least one person. Provide at least one male employee for heavy lifting, repairs, maintenance, and janitor work. Assign someone the responsibility of driving and running errands. And don't forget qualified administrative and office staff, especially if you, the administrator, are personally involved with nursing procedures.

When considering staff planning always include yourself and members of your family. They are contributing factors to your own financial needs whether they are actively employed or not. And in planning, fill in your own responsibility last, using yourself as a cushion or flexibility factor. You are one person who can work more than eight hours and can fill in on various jobs.

Don't forget, for economy of staffing it will be necessary for you to use the various types of nursing personnel in their proper functions. "Don't waste talent on work that does not require talent." For example, using an R.N. or L.P.N. for cleaning duties or expecting them to do work which any aide can perform is undesirable. You can hire someone much cheaper than an R.N. to do this type of work. On the other hand, an R.N. must not expect to do only medications, charts, treatments, and assist the doctors; she may also be asked to assist with more difficult nursing duties. You can make a mistake in hiring too many top-level personnel, as well as too few.

After you have done your best planning, you will need to evaluate it. Group the assignments according to geographical and plant location, as well as to the amount and type of work to be done. If your present staff is overworked, you will need to increase it. If employees have too little to do, delay for a while filling the next vacancy or discuss the problem with all of them and ask if some would like to take an extra day off so all can be kept on the payroll. Analyze work procedures and make use of labor-saving devices and movements. And at all times try to divide the work load evenly among all staff members.

RECRUITMENT

Recruitment and selection of the necessary staff is the next step. Naturally, we are all looking for the "ideal employee," the one who will do everything just the way we want it done for a very reasonable salary. Unfortunately, not enough of these employees are available. Some of the important qualifications are: dependability, basic good character, physical ability to do hard work (let's face it—it isn't easy work), cleanliness and neatness, common sense to meet emergencies and special situations, interest in people (especially the elderly), and a personality in harmony with those of other employees. Some personnel must also have supervisory ability. As said before, not all employees will have all of these qualifications. Usually, individual ability must be determined by trial and error. It is often necessary to hire inexperienced people and train them. This is frequently simpler than hiring the so-called "experienced" people who have to "unlearn" before they can "relearn."

There is a difference of opinion as to the hiring of young or old employees. Younger people have more vitality and adaptability, while older ones are more experienced and can meet emergencies better. Perhaps the best procedure would be to maintain a balance between the two. Some part-time employees will be needed, whether to assist during the peak hours of the day or to relieve regular employees on days off and during vacations. Some handicapped or hard-to-place persons may fit into your work situation. Here, adequate screening, investigation, and counseling will be extremely important.

How do you attract applicants? First of all, you must pay salaries and offer benefits which are attractive. Frequently, it is benefits and not salary which may gain or lose a prospective employee. Define the philosophy and standards of care which your home provides. People like to work for a good organization, so the more you can do to elevate the standards in your own home, the more status and prestige you will have to offer an employee. Your public relations in the community will say as much for you, as will your present employees. They can encourage and recruit new applicants for you.

Friends and contacts in outside agencies, trades, or professions may also refer applicants. Work with the personnel office of your local hospital. Do not overbid but keep salaries and benefits in line with theirs. Don't be afraid to hunt for applicants rather than wait for them to find you. You may locate more good applicants this way than by waiting for the desperate ones to call you. Advertise in your local paper or on institution bulletin boards. Also use the professional placement agencies and state employment offices. Do everything possible to build up the status of the position being filled. The type of dedicated employee we need is looking for a position which provides more job satisfaction than just his monthly pay check.

Many nurses, and other individuals, fail to see the challenges and opportunities offered in caring for the aged. Much of this is due to the publicity given substandard homes, with which, unfortunately, the good homes are grouped. So that nurses may know of these opportunities, I have long advocated that a portion of their professional nursing training be spent in nursing homes. At least invite your hospital to bring their senior students out for a field trip. After their tour, serve refreshments and make yourself available for answering questions.

I am happy to say that our home was one of the first of two approved by the State Office of Vocational Education and the Department of Registration and Education for a two-week training period for practical nursing students. These students are trained in the home for two weeks, 40 hours per week. During this period they are paid $4 per day. They are allowed to care for three patients each day, but they aren't to replace regular employees. They are in the home to learn, and their training includes four hours of classroom or ward teaching each week in the following departments: two hours in rehabilitative nursing, two hours in the activity program, one hour in office management, one hour in purchasing, one hour in dietary, and one hour in a study of the role of the nursing home in the health complex.

Although none of these L.P.N.'s are employed by our home, some of them have entered the nursing home field, and I am sure all of them profited from the experience they received in our facility. You, too, can encourage visits of such groups in your area to acquaint them with what our profession is doing, because many student nurses have no idea what nursing homes are really like.

Develop a definite system for screening and interviewing applicants. The application blank should supply much of the necessary information which can be discussed with the applicant and details clarified. In addition to getting information from the applicant, you will need to reveal to her a picture of your home by showing her around in person. A clear, definite understanding as to pay scale, working conditions, and house rules should be achieved at this interview. Job specifications and work routines are included at this time. Checking on references, especially with past employers, assists greatly in evaluating the applicant. If the nursing supervisor or another supervisory person will be dealing directly with the applicant, you may wish this person to interview her. Also, many homes now follow the practice of hiring employees for a probationary period of a specified length of time. In most states it is required that everyone have a preemployment physical examination. Don't neglect this because without it, injuries sustained prior to employment may become the basis for claims and law suits.

Personnel policies, formerly thought necessary to only large companies, are now becoming essential in nursing homes. Every well-run organization should have an established set of policies governing the conditions under which employees work and defining their rights and responsibilities. It is not enough that these policies be understood—they should be in printed form. This brochure should be given a new employee immediately and reviewed regularly at staff meetings. The aims and ideals of the home should be spelled out in this brochure. There should be sections on salaries, social security, fringe benefits, holiday pay, vacation pay, and pay dates. Also included should be information on coffee breaks and meal hours, standards of conduct and appearance, explanations of "chain of command," and criteria by which increases in pay are judged.

Personnel policies need not be lengthy or boring, but should be complete and consistent—a ready reference for old and new employees. One of the important factors which should be included and frequently is neglected is the part an employee personally plays in the public relations of your nursing home.

The residents are the objective of our service. Our prime goal is to give the best service possible. How we care for our residents determines the quality of our service; therefore, each employee must do all he can to keep them as happy and comfortable as possible. Kindness, love, cleanliness, and patience are four things that are necessary in caring for these people.

Employees should make relatives and friends feel welcome. A smile and a friendly "come back again" will go a long way toward this.

As soon as a doctor arrives he should be put in touch with the person in charge. He is a busy man and should be assisted in every way possible. The nurse in charge should accompany him to visit his patients and see that he has whatever he needs to care for them. She should ask questions that will help to provide better care and see that he writes orders on the charts and signs all previous orders that need his signature. He should be offered a cup of coffee or other refreshment. If he hasn't been through the nursing home to see the services offered, we should offer to show him through and try to explain our services and our philosophy of patient care.

Everyone should be willing to help a fellow worker to provide the best care possible for our residents. Friendliness is important, but we should not let overfamiliarity interfere with the work routine. If there is a rift or gripe between workers, the persons being cared for become aware that something is wrong and get uneasy and upset.

Good public relations is everybody's business. If employees enjoy their work, they should be public relations minded and tell their many friends about the good care that is being given the patients. They should be ever-ready to tell their physician, dentist, milkman, service station attendant, banker, laundryman, mailman, neighbors, friends, and relatives about the many good things that are happening where they work.

The only impression some people get of your home is how the telephone is answered and how phone calls are handled. Good telephone manners are very important. By being friendly, by having a smile in one's voice, and by offering to help or give the right information, much can be done to give a good impression of your home.

Unless these points are emphasized and included in your personnel policies the employee may not realize the important role she plays in your public relations.

The first few days on the job are crucial in the orientation and proper motivation of any new employee. She will already be under great tension, so your first objective must be to put her at ease. This can most readily be done by being pleasant and friendly. Show her how to record her time and introduce her to her co-workers and to patients. You will need to orient her to the physical plant again, particularly the area in which she will be working. Tell her as much about the routines as possible. Don't forget to show her the time schedule, explain coffee breaks and lunch hours, explain such forms as requisition and charge-out slips, the ever important B.M. chart, the suggestion box, and parking regulations. Residents, visitors, and employees may drop unsigned suggestions in the suggestion box; later these should be discussed at staff meetings.

Many nursing home employees are trained on the job and so will be learning at the bedside rather than in the classroom. Proper instruction is necessary, with recurring demonstration and supervision until mastery. Emphasize from the beginning that she will be expected to carry on as she has been taught even when not under close supervision. Emphasize the responsibilities during various shifts, stating that on each shift specific duties must be performed during assigned hours.

Since nursing homes usually have reasonably small staffs and a relatively stable census, most of us strive for a "large happy family" type of working arrangement. Unfortunately, the new employee is sometimes not welcomed as warmly as we would like, even if we are desperate for help, so proper attitudes toward a new employee will aid our regular employees to accept her.

Proper attitude is most important and must radiate from everyone—administrator down to yardman. This is especially true in this day of rehabilitative nursing, where all must learn the importance of helping the patient to help himself, rather than doing things for him. Detailed and repeated explanations added to many introductions cannot be remembered easily. At the end of the first day the new employee is apt to be thoroughly confused. It is well to remind her to feel free to ask questions at any time.

"Once teaching" of a new employee is never enough. There must be constant supervision and reteaching. This job is much simpler if you have succeeded in enlisting the "hearts" of your staff members along with their "hands." If each employee is truly interested in giving her patients the best possible care and really wants to do a good job, this will show in her day-to-day work. But even the best group of employees needs supervision. Lack of supervision leads to confusion, and confusion means time lost and a lower grade of nursing care given.

It is necessary to have time schedules and assignment sheets. Make the time sheets out a month in advance. Allow for special requests even though it may require changing for the unexpected. Rotate weekends and holidays. We have found that assigning patients and work loads by groups and rotating them on a monthly basis has been quite satisfactory.

Much time is spent in explaining to an employee how you want things done. To eliminate confusion write out work steps definitely and explicitly. And then put your directions in manual form. The improvement of service which can come from such a manual is enormous. Here, too, work routines and job specifications are important. Sometimes it is impossible (or impractical) to work out such routines. In such cases it may be better to tell the girls what you expect and then let them work out their own routines. At least, enlist the aid of your staff in developing work routines. Trust the intelligence of your employees, but don't expect miracles. Do recognize and adopt good methods which an employee discovers.

Other suggestions for closer supervision are:

1. Do the task yourself so you are able to orient the new employee to the work.

2. Work all shifts occasionally so you know the around-the-clock problems.

3. Supervise personally by conference, finding out what employees want and why, how a task is being done and why, etc.

4. Do some supervision by means of written reports.

5. Delegate some supervisory duties to the R.N., head cook, etc.

6. Have new employees work near experienced ones.

7. Criticize and correct when something is done incorrectly. Constructive criticism is essential, but don't forget to praise when praise is deserved.

8. Be available for explanation or help when needed.

9. Keep channels of communication open, such as where you are and when you will return.

MOTIVATION

Labor turnover is expensive financially and emotionally; it affects not only you but the rest of the staff and the patients. Motivation is getting people to want to do their work. The amount of salary offered is one factor but it isn't everything. Fringe benefits are also important. Helping the employees to feel pride in their positions is a very important nonmonetary reward. A little bit of praise goes a long way. Recognition of faithful service can also be verbal or can be shown by parties and get-togethers, service pins, shoulder patches and emblems, or a promotion to more responsibility.

IN-SERVICE TRAINING

Employees are usually happier when they have an opportunity to learn. This can be accomplished through in-service education, classroom teaching, Red Cross courses, and monthly county nursing home educational programs. Job satisfaction depends also on the employer-employee relationship. We must radiate friendship and happiness, express appreciation and personal interest, and be considerate of each other's feelings. We cannot be too aloof and unapproachable; nor can we be buddy-buddy. We must learn to criticize, correct, and to say "no" when necessary. Psychological reward from the job is of equal importance to the monetary reward.

In-service education is an invaluable method of teaching. In some cases this means formal meetings; in other cases it may be more an impromptu, spontaneous discussion between two or three employees. State standards are beginning to require this education as a part of the regular program in your home. These meetings may involve the entire staff or only certain specified groups. A warm, friendly atmosphere should prevail—possibly preceded by a warm-up coffee session. The range of topics to be discussed is vast, the primary topic being, of course, the individual resident—his health, behavior, and personality. In any case, staff meetings result in more efficient management, better patient care, increased communication, and improved staff morale.

EVALUATION OF EMPLOYEES

Each administrator regularly evaluates his employees. More often than not, this is done in a fleeting manner in his own mind. It should also be done more formally, with a written evaluation followed by a conference and discussion between the employee and the evaluator. No employee is all good or all bad, but you must set up some consistent standards by which to judge them. Some points to be considered are quality of work, speed and amount of work, job knowledge, industriousness, reaction to emergencies and unusual situations, appearance and personality, as well as stability and dependability. You will need a checklist of the points to be considered. Many types of printed forms are now available. Naturally, the person doing the evaluation will need to supervise closely enough to accurately form these opinions. Regardless of how you evaluate your workers, it is necessary that you have job descriptions, work routines, and good methods of communications so that each worker knows exactly what is expected of her. Set high (but not unreasonable) standards and expect conformity. An employee who knows what she is expected to do, and why she is expected to do it, exercises a large amount of self-discipline, simplifying your problem.

DISCIPLINE

Inevitably, at times you will be required to act as a "buffer" when your supervisory person has an employee who must be disciplined. Never reprimand an employee in public. Always be fair, consistent, and considerate; however, certain improper actions call for dismissal. I consider any of the following in this category:

1. abusive and inconsiderate treatment of patients

2. willful destruction of property
3. stealing, deceit, or other dishonesty
4. reporting to work under the influence of liquor, or the use of liquor on the premises
5. insubordination or failure to carry out instructions and job assignments issued by supervisors
6. inefficiency
7. acts disregarding established personnel procedures
8. excessive absences, or abuse of a leave of absence
9. repeated garnishments of the employee's wages
10. accepting monetary gratuities or gifts from patients or visitors
11. punching another employee's time card
12. gossiping about patients

If you must discharge someone, do it as tactfully as possible. Written accounts of oral conferences, kept on file, are invaluable for showing that a dismissal was justified. Don't be too hasty but, when strict action is indicated, it is your responsibility to stand firm. The ultimate control over all actions must remain in your hands.

It would be impossible to discuss all the aspects of personnel management thoroughly at this time. Even the best personnel management will be in vain unless you provide your employees with proper equipment in good repair and adequate supplies to enable them to do their job well. This combination should result in a well-trained, highly motivated, and contented staff which will reflect a well-run nursing home.

HOME MANAGEMENT

In managing a home one's first thoughts must be directed toward aims and goals.

Do you wish to serve the need of a small or large community? Do you wish to serve the patient who requires post-hospital care before going home, along with your long-term patient? Do you wish to serve the young as well as the aging patient? Are the people in this community accustomed to spacious living or large-city apartment living? Will they want outside activities? People do not necessarily wish to change their customs just because they are aging or infirmed from a chronic disease. These are but a few of the factors influencing your choice of land and location.

Once you decide on the area where you want to locate it is necessary to determine the feasibility of the project before negotiating for the property. Will the community support the project? Is there a need? Today there are areas that may be overbuilding just because someone wants to stay in a particular location. Such an area isn't always the area that has a need for your program or can support it.

How do you determine a need? Personally, I don't have much confidence in the formulas presently being used for determining nursing home needs for those who are 65 years of age and older. Just because people are over that age doesn't mean they are ill and in need of nursing care. However, much advice and assistance can be obtained by talking with county, regional, and/or state health department personnel.

THE PROBLEM OF LOCATION

Check with the paying agency to see if their rates are commensurate with the programs you are planning and if there are a number of recipients on their rolls who are in hospitals and can be transferred to a facility such as the one you are planning. Check with the local hospitals regarding their average occupancy, as well as the number of patients who are occupying beds that could be used for the acutely ill who are waiting to be admitted. Visit with the physicians in the community; determine if they understand the role of the nursing home in the health and medical care facility complex. Talk with representatives of the visiting nurse association, the home care program, and nursing home administrators.

Once you are satisfied there is a need and you know whom you are going to serve, begin your search for the property. If you have decided to serve the short-term convalescent as well as the long-term resident it is desirable, in my mind, to locate near a hospital which is convenient for the patient and which gives him the assurance that laboratory, X-ray, and emergency services are nearby. The services of his own physician in making regular as well as emergency calls on the way to and from the hospital or office and home should be readily available.

Transportation to a community hospital is usually good, therefore such a location would improve your opportunities for obtaining employees, as well as encouraging visitors for your patients, which is essential.

The cost that may be involved in purchasing such a location may, in the long run, be less than the cost of a home that is lower-priced initially. It may mean that you will get more referrals from physicians since they like to keep their patients, and the patients like to keep their family doctors. Physicians are very busy and it is not always possible to travel miles to see one or two patients.

Of course, it is usually an area such as this that presents zoning problems, but this resistance must be overcome for the benefit of those we serve. They are entitled to nice surroundings, a good neighborhood, convenient transportation for patient, family, physician, and employees. It is wise to start cultivating your future neighbors as early as possible and to acquaint them with the function of your facility before the zoning hearing is due.

How much land do you need? Remember to include parking areas for employees, families, physicians, volunteers, salesmen, and others; avoid a parking menace on the street which would provoke your neighbors. Build goodwill, thereby receiving referrals from your families and physicians by having a restricted parking area for them.

Spacious grounds not only create a beautiful setting, but also may encourage gardening. Your architect will help in getting the most from your land, with adequate space for your plant, plus expansion if this is part of your planning. It is wise to keep in mind that the nursing home field is on a threshold of a new era. With the rapid increase in hospital costs and the accreditation of nursing homes, insurance companies and third-party payors are becoming interested in good patient care at the right cost.

If you expect to have the fullest cooperation with your state agencies, the site should be approved by them, and in my state, the plans must be approved by the architect of the State Department of Public Health before you are allowed to "put a spade in the ground."

However, much earlier than this stage (but immediately after the location has been settled), it is necessary to engage the services of a competent architect, at least on a preliminary basis. Inasmuch as most state health departments require submission of plans prior to construction, it is well to have a preliminary visit with your health department and to present a rough sketch of what is being proposed. Most architects will prepare such sketches for a nominal fee. It is wise to discuss the project with the state health department before embarking upon the building program because it can often provide additional facts and figures that will be helpful in evaluating the merits of the proposed location.

Conformity with all the standards from the start of a project will certainly make for better public relations with licensing authorities and public safety bureaus. Rules and regulations have been made because of failures on the part of individuals to do everything in their power for the safety and well-being of human beings. So when something happens that is disastrous, or just plain uncomfortable, a new rule or regulation is established and enforced. A large percentage of the building codes deal with fire prevention and a small percentage with other safeguards. Before actual construction is started, it is advisable to have the Bureau of Insurance check the plans since their recommendations may affect the cost of insurance.

PLANNING THE BUILDING

Now that you have your architect, land, and approval of site, it is time to give even more consideration to the next phase of your project—planning your building. Any mistakes made in this phase are something you live with the rest of your life and they can also be costly. At times we have a tendency to cut corners, thinking about the initial cost, when, if time were taken to figure additional costs in order to have a more functional building, it might amount to only a few cents a day more (over the 20-year mortgage period) compared with a dollars-per-day cost in labor or time. Discuss your plans with knowledgeable people, such as a nurse who has been directing nursing in a nursing home, or a dietitian.

When you know what you want, then begin searching for your financing. When you approach a finance house, it is fruitful to have your plans formulated and a projected operating statement available. Approach them in a businesslike manner. Know how much money you want, for how long, and the interest you are willing to pay.

After financing is obtained, you are ready to select your builder and begin construction. A one-floor building is preferable, without steps or threshold plates, for this is best suited to the needs of patients in wheelchairs and on crutches. It also reduces the work and travel time of the staff.

The interior arrangement is important for the safety and comfort of the patients. A cheerful and pleasant atmosphere is conducive to the general well-being of the residents, workers, and visitors.

Long-term residents, particularly the aged, are likely to take to their beds and generally retreat from the world if they are permitted to do so. It is just too much trouble to dress and move around, even when their physical capacity permits it. In this they are too often abetted by attendants who find it easier to care for patients in their beds rather than go through the physical and psychological struggle of getting them up. It is to avoid this tendency to withdraw that the recreation area, therapy room, dining room, nurses' station, lobby, and administrative offices should be centrally located.

The administrator and charge nurse will have better control of activities in all these areas and can encourage more active participation by the residents.

The living room and lobby area should be used by residents and visitors at any reasonable hour. This gives the residents an opportunity to visit with each other and to associate with the many people who come into the home. Television placed in this area is a valuable asset. This should be a cheerful room with sturdy furniture well arranged so that there is room for those with walkers, canes, and wheelchairs to move around with ease. The sofas and chairs should have wide arms, rather firm seats, and be neither so deep or low as to strain the joints and backs of the patients.

A few tables and lamps are essential in this area. Providing plants, vines, fish, and birds will create a homelike atmosphere and friendliness, and will help meet the residents' needs for affection and emotional security.

I do not agree with some authorities that this family room should be at the rear of the building because of the effect it has on families who are looking for a place for their loved ones. It is time we change the image of the aging and infirmed. I believe having this room near the entrance has been more an asset than not. Really, how many families want their loved ones hidden?

Bedrooms should be large enough to accommodate essential furniture, plus wheelchair, cane, and walker passage. Each resident should have a closet and drawer space, a bedside table, an overbed table, and easy and straight chairs for his own use. Toilets and lavatories should be convenient to encourage self-help and the retraining activities of daily living. Provide screening devices in semi-private or ward rooms, remembering to protect the dignity of individuals. Call buttons, proper lighting, ventilation, and heat are important. The windows should be low enough to permit a resident to see outside whether in bed or in a chair. The decor of the residents' rooms is as essential as in the service or entrance areas. Soft colors are best for the walls, with the use of colorful drapes, spreads, and chair coverings to provide a harmonizing effect.

The desirable square footage for bedrooms should be approximately 125 in a multiple bedroom and 100 in a single room. The beds should be 4 feet apart, and 3 feet from adjacent walls, closets, and other fixtures. Doors to residents' rooms should be 3 feet, 8 inches wide; 3 feet wide for toilet-room doors.

It is desirable to have at least one-half the beds the hi-low type with the other half of stationary height. I prefer the beds to be 23 inches high instead of the regular 19 inches because this height permits residents to get in and out of bed more comfortably. The regular dormitory bed is too low for stiff joints.

We have provided half the rooms in our home with lavatories in each room for more efficiency, making it possible for all four residents to be busy at the same time. Many times this has been a selling point for relatives. They don't mind if mother or dad has to share a toilet with three others, but they object to their sharing a lavatory.

BATHROOMS AND BATHING TECHNIQUES

The toilet room should be large enough for a wheelchair, and the toilet should be equipped with grab bars. A bedpan washer at each stool is a time-saver for the nurses.

Bathrooms should be centrally located and screened properly if more than one bathing facility is in one room. Most of the people entering nursing homes need supervised bathing; therefore, to discourage accidents, a limited number of private baths are provided. In the bathrooms an elevated, regular and collapsible tub, and a shower stall are essential, for many residents prefer specific bathing techniques. By providing for their wishes, it is easier on bath days to get the job done without fuss and without forcing our own desires on them. The water temperature should be controlled so as not to burn the residents. The aged are susceptible to burns. Emergency call buttons should be provided in all toilet-and bathrooms.

THE DINING AREA

The dining room should be well lighted and cheery, located near the kitchen, and equidistant from all bedroom wings. Remember the wheelchair patients who will be coming into the dining area and provide a room large enough to allow their passage. A small table accommodating four is desirable for grouping individuals who are congenial, as well as taking care of the untidy eaters and those on special diets. If you are planning a self-help and rehabilitative nursing program, you will need room for about 75 to 90 per cent of your occupancy.

A dining room can double as an additional recreation room for large group meetings, such as chapel services, movies, or speakers. It can also be used for educational staff conferences. Beds or other pieces of equipment for demonstration purposes can be moved around in this room and there will be adequate sitting room for all staff members.

RECREATION AND MULTIPURPOSE AREA

Your recreation room can be used for problem eaters, and for a second living room. This area should have worktables, chairs of sturdy construction which will not overturn easily, television, a record player, sink, refrigerator, and a hot plate, so that games, crafts, and refreshments can be encouraged for all. Cabinets and shelves for storage of games, books, and magazines should be provided, and a display rack for crafts is needed.

In the physical therapy room provide parallel bars, exercise pulley board and mat, treatment tables, and steps. All this equipment can be made in your own shop with little expense. Have plumbing installed, in case you find the physicians requesting a hip or limb tank at a later date. This room usually has minimum equipment for a limited type program because we are not trying to duplicate services offered in the hospitals and can only carry on therapy that can be done by an aide and nurses under the direction of a physical therapist and orders of the physician.

The multipurpose room can serve as a beauty and barber shop, treatment and examining room, and you can utilize the same chair for podiatry services and dental services with a portable dental kit. These can be scheduled at different times and on different days.

Provide a staff dining room and lounge area so that employees have a place to relax and call their own. This is essential in making them happier, for we cannot operate well without contented employees.

NURSING STATION

The nursing station, which is the nerve center of every nursing home, should be well arranged with proper equipment and supplies, if it is to serve us properly. Clean and soiled work areas are a necessity and should be close to the nursing station. Provide a communication system that will eliminate many trips a day to find out why the call light is on and one that assures that patient needs will be taken care of promptly. Provide charts and chart racks for record keeping, which is vitally important to the resident, physician, nurses, and the home-owners. Telephones must be available in all critical areas.

A refrigerator and a locked medicine cabinet for drugs, and a storage area with a small autoclave and utensil sterilizer should be available at or near the nurses' station. It may also be necessary to provide substations in bedroom wings to save steps. It is suggested that for every forty beds a nurses' station is desirable.

ADMINISTRATIVE OFFICES

Well-planned administrative and business offices are essential in all homes if business is to be conducted properly. It is becoming more and more essential that the administrator have an accurate accounting of the business at all times. It is important to know how each area or department is running in cost and if there is any inefficiency. So if these two administrative offices adjoin, this offers an opportunity to review records quickly, at any time of day.

KITCHEN AREA

Kitchen planning needs to be centered around meal planning, nutrition, sanitation, work convenience, and proper equipment. The walls and floors must withstand much scrubbing and hard wear. They must be easily cleaned. Controlling cooking odors and heat requires an adequate number of windows, fans, and exhaust fans.

The kitchen should be located so that it can easily serve residents' bedrooms, the central dining area, and the staff dining room. It should be near the service entrance, storerooms, deep freeze, and walk-in cooler.

Equipment such as ranges, refrigerators, toasters, coffee makers, and garbage disposals should be heavy-duty, so that they will withstand the constant use. The sizes of pots and pans should be standardized to the sizes of ovens and shelves in order to better utilize all equipment.

I am finally convinced, after great resistance, that a steam table is worth every dollar it costs. It is a time-saver for the cook, and it keeps the food palatable from the time the first tray is served until the last staff member is served.

Plan your areas of preparation, cooking, baking, serving, and dishwashing with time-saving in mind. Plenty of refrigeration will be needed in the kitchen, along with counter space, storage areas, and sinks to provide a convenience to your cooks and kitchen helpers, and to make for desirable working conditions. Also, a hand sink must be located in the kitchen for the kitchen employees. Adequate storage areas are needed in all phases of operations but don't cut yourself short on space for kitchen, general, and maintenance storage.

LAUNDRY FACILITIES

To do or not to do your laundry on the premises is a highly controversial subject. Again, much depends on your locale. Is there a commercial laundry available to give you good service, and is it competitive in its price? If laundry is done commercially, you need to provide for a soiled linen area, located conveniently for pickup. Also needed will be a clean-linen area for delivery, counting, and sorting. The size of these two rooms will be determined by the amount of linen used, frequency of pickup and delivery. It will be necessary to provide a small laundry unit for personal laundry, and also for processing linen used by incontinent patients either before it is sent to the laundry or on weekends when there is no delivery.

If the laundry is to be done on the premises, select the proper equipment. From personal experience, I would recommend commercial laundry equipment even in a small home of fifteen or sixteen beds. I have found it to be false economy to attempt to get along with household appliances. Constant repairs are needed, machines are running day and night, and it is necessary for the nursing personnel to do laundry. Nursing personnel should do only nursing, and their services are usually more costly than those of domestics.

The laundry should be located in the service area away from the patients and food, and manned by a person hired specifically for the job, and not one involved also with cooking or nursing. The room needs plenty of ventilation because the heat from the ironer and dryer is quite intense. It should be roomy and easily cleaned in order to be kept pleasant and attractive. The machinery should be geared to the size of your facility. Any reputable manufacturer will consult with you as to what is adequate. Talk with more than one representative.

Dirty linen should not be allowed to accumulate for any period of time if you expect to control odors. Feces in linen should be washed out in the soiled-linen utility room before being sent to the laundry or placed into a hamper. Precaution must be used to keep contamination at a minimum. Laundry employees must be taught the dangers of cross-infection and how to prevent it in their department. It is necessary to furnish this area with the proper carts for transporting soiled and clean linen.

All residents' articles should be properly marked, washed, starched, and ironed as carefully and properly as you would your own washables. Mending is a function of the laundry department. The house linen must be kept white and in good repair. All soaps and detergents do not work the same in different localities; therefore, it is sometimes necessary to experiment or have someone analyze the water for mineral content if your linen acquires the "tell-tale gray."

Iron only the pieces that require ironing. We find that by removing contour and draw sheets before entirely dry, folding, and stacking, they do not require ironing. Pillowcases, sheets, and gowns are ironed with the ironer. Residents' clothes are hand-ironed. The balance is folded and stacked until used.

Put clothes away properly. Nothing is quite as upsetting to a family as to have mother's gown on someone else, or to be unable to find it because it is in someone else's drawer. Keep extra linens under lock and key to discourage temptation. I believe more linen than food disappears from all types of institutions.

In planning the boiler room, adequate heating to maintain approximately 75 degrees temperature, and sufficient hot water for rooms, cooking, and laundry must be considered. The mechanical or boiler room may also have a workbench to handle general repairs, and an incinerator to facilitate the disposal of trash and waste that cannot be processed in the garbage disposal.

Other areas needed are public rest rooms and employees' rest rooms for both sexes; a public telephone booth, low enough and in a large enough area for wheelchair patients; and a drinking fountain accessible to patients and nurses. The ideal height is 36 inches.

Corridors should be at least 7 feet wide, preferably 8 feet, with handrails on both sides about 3 feet from the floor. At least one janitor closet, centrally located to all areas, is needed.

GOOD HOUSEKEEPING

The physical plant must be kept clean, sanitary, and odor-free. Your good public image is dependent on good housekeeping. It is most important to the safety, health, and morale of patients and staff. Have as organized a system in your housekeeping department as you would in the nursing or dietary departments.

The housekeeper must see that corridors, offices, lobbies, service areas, patients' rooms, and bathrooms are dusted, swept, mopped regularly and frequently, and waxed as needed. The furniture must be kept clean and polished and the wastebaskets emptied regularly. The housekeeper may also assist the maintenance department by reporting the need for repair and/or replacement.

It is equally desirable to provide this department, as well as the others, with adequate supplies and equipment. Keep in mind the person doing the cleaning and polishing. If this employee is a woman, don't supply the largest mop, pails, or polisher you can find. Without proper equipment it is very discouraging to be unable to complete such chores regularly and on schedule.

SAFETY MEASURES

We, as nursing home administrators, have a moral, as well as a legal responsibility to avoid the possibility of accidental deaths and injuries among our residents, employees, and visitors. Therefore, we must construct, equip, and manage our facilities so that they will not constitute a hazard to anyone.

Fire safety is of grave concern to all of us. In planning we must determine whether enough water is available, whether the fire department is adequate, and whether we need a sprinkler and/or fire detection system, fire-resistant materials, and wire glass. Smoke detectors will be more readily available in the next few years and they will respond more quickly than a notifier or sprinkler. A magnetic doorholder system in connection with the sound system is being developed.

Do not let trash, paint rags, mops, and like hazards accumulate. Regulate the smoking of residents, employees, and visitors. Proper types and adequate numbers of fire extinguishers should be placed advantageously. It is as important to have your personnel trained for fire safety, evacuation, and disaster planning as it is to take all the precautions.

The local fire-fighting men should be acquainted with your physical plant layout, type of construction, and location of rooms. They should visit once or twice a year to keep the plant layout in their minds, and to keep the staff conscious of the necessity to be constantly on the alert for fire detection. The local firemen are usually available for staff training on the use of fire extinguishers, methods of preventing the spread of fire, and an evacuation program.

We need to be constantly aware of many other safety factors: side rails on beds, grab bars at toilet and bath areas, nonskid floor surfaces, brakes on wheelchairs, handrails in hallways, good electrical repair, poisonous drugs stored separately from other drugs, precautions in drug giving and drug storing, proper storage and administration of oxygen, the removing of obstacles and obstructions, and keeping facilities well lighted. We could explore many other areas such as safety in the laundry and kitchen, and in housekeeping procedures, but it is possible to get much help from knowledgeable people in your own community who will assist you with these safety or hazard factors.

MAINTENANCE AND REPAIR

An organized maintenance program will save time and money, and it will keep the building and items of equipment in serviceable condition or else return them to serviceable condition.

Preventive maintenance will prevent breakdown and extend the life of the equipment and plant. Whoever is responsible for your preventive work must be well acquainted with the specifications of every piece of equipment in the home so that he will know their working parts. It is just as disastrous to supply an overabundance of oil or grease to a valve as it is to ignore it altogether. There should be a regular work schedule for cleaning and oiling motors, checking and fixing plumbing, furnaces, refrigerators, freezers, gas and electrical appliances, and laundry equipment. A record card should be kept for each piece of major equipment, showing identification data, location in the home, plate data, cost, date purchased, inspection and service instructions.

Repair and preserve furniture regularly and at intervals when needed. A little "doing" while the need is still minor may save you the price of a new piece of equipment. Your nursing-care equipment such as canes, crutches, walkers, and wheelchairs need periodical oiling, cleaning, adjusting, and painting. To encourage maintenance men to do a good job you must furnish adequate tools and a place for them to call their own so that they will perform at their highest level.

Some outside storage may be necessary for things that will be needed in the upkeep of the property. Remember that your yard and building exterior are the "picture" you present to the public.

This has been a bird's-eye view of management in which we have reviewed land and locations, building standards, management of building projects, maintenance, repair, safety, and how to plan and arrange your various rooms and service areas. On paper it may sound simple and elementary but, truly, a nursing and/or retirement home administrator must be a knowledgeable person in many fields.

REFERENCES

1. Whale, Guy, Jr., "Six Steps to Better Hospital Purchasing." *Hospitals,* 37: 53–55, January 1, 1963.
2. Borlin, Harlan F., "The Ethics of Purchasing." *Professional Nursing Homes,* 4:8:28, August 1962.
3. "How Do You Buy the Small Supply." *Institutions Magazine,* pp. 56–58, March 1963.
4. Gerletti, John D. *et al. Nursing Home Administration.* Downey, Calif.: Attending Staff Association, 1961.
5. Proud, Dorothy M., *Buying Food for Your Nursing Home.* Ithaca, N.Y.: New York State Extension Service, Cornell University, May 1961.
6. Nelson, K. R., Jr., "An Evaluation Program for Aides." *Professional Nursing Homes,* 3:6:13, June 1961.

7. Shore, Herbert, "You Can Have More Effective Staff Meetings." *Professional Nursing Homes,* 4:11:30, November 1962.
8. Baltz, Florence L., "Nursing Care: Its Importance, Its Problems." *Hospital Progress,* June 1960.
9. ———, "How To Staff a 20-Bed Nursing Home." *The Modern Hospital,* 98:6:16, June 1962.
10. Bainum, Robert, "So You're Going To Build a Nursing Home." *Nursing Homes,* Part I, 12:1:5–7; 18–21, January 1963 and Part II, 12:2:18–21, February 1963.
11. "Long Term Care Facilities Hospitals." *Journal American Hospital Association,* 37:3:48, March 1, 1963.
12. Nicholson, Edna, *Planning New Institutional Facilities for Long Term Care.* New York: Putnam, 1956.
13. Williams, R. C. *et al., Nursing Home Management.* New York: McGraw-Hill, 1959.
14. "Long Term Care: A Backdrop of Facts." *Journal American Hospital Association,* 36:41, January 16, 1962.
15. Williams, Helen, "Plan To Be Safe." *Nursing Homes,* 11:11:5–6; 22–23, 1962.
16. Mustin, George, "If You Want To Build a Better Nursing Home." *Professional Nursing Home,* 5:1:18, January 1963.
17. "This Nursing Home Keeps Patients Busy." *The Modern Hospital,* 98:5:91–93, May 1962.

Chapter 16

Building an Adequate Insurance Program

EMMETT J. VAUGHAN, *Ph.D.*

In recent years a large portion of the public has become better educated and informed concerning insurance as a product. This has been especially true in the business world. As the outlay for insurance premiums has come to be a more and more significant item in the budgets of firms, an increasing amount of attention has been devoted to this expenditure. Price consciousness on the part of insurance buyers has led to a greater interest in the matters of proper coverages and total costs.

Many firms have taken a scientific approach to the problem of insurance buying, and a large number of firms now have highly trained people who specialize in risk management and insurance buying. In some cases this is a full-time job for one person, or even for a special department in the company. Because they are responsible for the whole program of risk management and purchasing insurance for the firm, these people are known as "risk managers."

In the nursing and retirement home, the risk manager is probably the same person that manages everything else, the administrator. He is the person who makes the decision as to what kind of insurance should be purchased, how much, and from whom. His task as the risk manager of the home is an extremely heavy burden, for it is a job that requires the utmost precision if loss is to be avoided. If the home is underinsured, it will suffer financially if a loss occurs. If, on the other hand, it is overinsured, the loss is just as real in terms of the premiums that should not have been spent, for the legal principle of indemnity states that the insured cannot collect more than the amount of his loss, regardless of the amount of insurance he has paid for.

Certainly, the risk manager needs all the help he can get. He may seek and receive help before making his decisions, but in the last analysis, risk management and the insurance program remain his burden. Unfortunately, the risk manager who most needs help, that is, the risk manager who is also the office manager, the personnel manager, and just about everything else, is the risk manager who is least likely to find himself advised by people who are genuinely interested in advising (as distinguished from selling), or who are capable of advising. For this reason, the administrator must understand and appreciate the aspects of risk management. He must know enough about risk management to recognize whether his advisors on the subject are any good. He must, in other words, know enough about risk management to know when he needs help, and be able to determine whether he is getting the kind of help he needs.

Insurance company representatives and agents can be very helpful in advising the risk manager, particularly with regard to the purchase of insurance. As you know, the insurance agent receives his commission for the service which he renders before and after the sale. The portion of your premium dollar which goes to compensate a competent agent advisor is well spent.

More than one hundred years ago, John Ruskin said, "There is hardly anything in this world that some man cannot make a little poorer and sell a little cheaper, and people who consider price only are this man's lawful prey." In some cases it may be possible to purchase insurance at reduced rates by eliminating the services of the agent and purchasing the coverage directly from a company, but before you make such a decision, make sure that you can do without the services of the agent. Companies which sell directly to the insured can in some cases provide pure protection at a reduced rate, but this reduced rate may entail a reduction in the services to which you have been accustomed. The greatest savings in premium dollars can be achieved by proper programming of the insurance coverages to meet the needs.

Basically, the responsibilities and functions of the agent are to work with the client in analyzing the insurable exposures and risks, and then to select the proper policy forms and to negotiate the program agreed upon in consultation with the insured. From time immemorial, professional agents have avoided the "shotgun" method of selling and have attempted to help the insured to view his insurance problem as a single problem, rather than as many separate individual problems.

The risk manager who does not have access to a competent agent advisor must of necessity make his own decisions regarding his insurance program, for it often takes a great deal of looking to find a good advisor.

THE RISKS YOU FACE

The risk manager must take certain basic steps in developing his insurance program. The first step is to determine exactly what the risks facing the home are. Second, a decision must be made as to which of these risks should be insured, which risks should be avoided, and which risks the home should do nothing about. Finally, insurance coverages should be obtained to transfer those risks which the home wishes to avoid.

In general, nursing and retirement homes face many of the same risks that confront the individual. In general too, we can classify these risks under four headings: death or disability; legal liability; loss of property; indirect loss.

DEATH OR DISABILITY

Premature death may cause serious loss to the home. If one individual in the organization makes a significant contribution to the success of the home, his death may be the equivalent of the death of the home. At the same time, if such an employee becomes disabled, the home may not only lose his services, but may be obligated to continue the salary of this disabled person.

LEGAL LIABILITY

As with individuals, the home may become liable to others for bodily injury or property damage. Actually, the possibility of such liability is much greater for a nursing or retirement home than for an individual, since the home is responsible for the activities of its employees, as well as for the services it performs. At one time there was a significant difference in the liability exposure of charitable institutions and profit-making ones, but this distinction has gradually disappeared, so that today the eleemosynary institution faces the same risk of being brought into court as a profit-making business.

Basically, there are four separate liability exposures: employer's liability and workmen's compensation; general liability; automobile liability; professional liability.

LOSS OF PROPERTY

The home also faces the risk of property damage or loss. Fire or other perils may destroy the building and the furnishings. Dishonest employees, as well as others, may steal from the firm.

INDIRECT LOSS

Another serious source of loss is indirect loss, which stems from the consequences of a direct loss. For example, a fire may damage property owned by the home. As a consequence, the home may be prevented from continuing operation, or it may be able to continue operations only by moving to a temporary location at considerable expense.

In addition to these, numerous other risks are present, and there are an almost unlimited number of insurance contracts available to protect against this equally unlimited number of hazards and exposures. It is self-evident that it would be impossible to insure against every conceivable loss. With the limited resources available that may be devoted to the purchase of insurance, the task becomes one of choosing among alternatives, and the risk manager needs some principle to guide him.

The first and foremost principle of risk management is that the probability that a loss may occur is less important than the possible size of the loss. Once a risk has been identified, its significance must be evaluated from the point of view of the size of the possible loss that could result, and not the probability that the loss may or may not occur. On the basis of this first principle, we derive the major working concept of risk management. The most important losses, or the risks that should be insured first, are those that would place the greatest burden on the assets of the home if that loss should occur. The relatively small loss that occurs with relative frequency is not a proper subject for insurance. The cost of such losses should be budgeted.

Bear in mind that the purpose of insurance is not that of eliminating all risks, large and small. An insurance contract is purposeful and meaningful when it is used to insure those risks and losses that are unpredictable, and only those that will involve the insured in a major financial catastrophe. An insured can pay for small losses himself without much financial difficulty. It is the relatively large loss—the one that would "put his back to the wall" financially if he did not have insurance—that should be insured.

On the basis of this principle, the losses that we should seek to avoid first are those that would work the greatest hardship on the home if they should occur. With this in mind, we can begin to construct an insurance program.

THE INSURANCE PROGRAM

The loss of a key man might well be a crucial blow to the home, and might mean the end of the home itself. For this reason, if such a person is a part of the organization, the program should begin with life insurance on this individual, in some amount that would permit the home to make the adjustment in the event his services were lost.

Once this has been taken care of, the loss that appears potentially the greatest is the liability exposure. It has no fixed limit. Obviously the maximum loss that can occur to the property of the home is limited by the value of that property. A lawsuit might well cost the home a judgment that is far greater than the value of the property itself.

It is important that each of the four basic categories of liability exposure be covered. The first, which includes the liability insurance to cover workers who are injured at work, can be covered by the standard Workmen's Compensation Policy with employer's liability. This coverage is required by law, so we begin with it as the basis of our liability coverage.

The general liability exposure consists of the potential liability to outsiders—to persons who are not employees and who are not patients. This exposure can be covered by one of several policies, the best of which is the Comprehensive General Liability Policy. This policy covers all of the liability exposures of the home except workmen's compensation, the automobile, and professional liability.

Automobiles are a serious source of liability, and probably the liability exposure that most people think of first. Most firms own automobiles. Even if they do not, there is need for automobile liability insurance. Employees often drive their automobiles or the cars of others in the course of their employment, and if they injure someone while doing so, the home can be held liable. Many risk managers who readily recognize the liability hazard of the vehicles owned by the home do not consider the liability exposure involved in the automobiles of employees. This risk is easily overlooked because the employer or administrator may not have an awareness that the employee is using the auto in the course of employment. This hazard can be covered by the non-ownership liability endorsement to the auto liability policy. As a matter of fact, the auto liability coverage can be included with the general liability coverage in one policy.

Professional liability insurance was originally called malpractice insurance. The liability exposure of a nursing or retirement home can and should be covered under a hospital liability policy. If the home has such a policy, the insurance company will defend all suits alleging malpractice, paying the entire cost of the defense, and, in addition, will pay any judgment assessed against the home, up to the limits of liability of the policy. If the administrator is a professional man who administers treatment of any kind, he, too, will need a professional liability policy, for the hospital liability policy does not cover the liability of any of the individuals who work in the home and who might be joined in a suit against the home. Likewise, the individual's liability policy does not cover the liability exposure of the insured as the proprietor or administrator of the home, nor does it cover the liability of the institution itself. So two or more professional liability policies are necessary. Incidentally, these contracts should be written in the same insurance company to avoid any disputes that might arise as to which policy applies in a given instance.

The hospital liability policy can be purchased as a separate contract, or, like automobile liability, it can be included in the Comprehensive General Liability-Automobile Liability policy. The latter is probably the better approach, for it combines all of the liability protection in one contract with one insurer.

We have not covered the subject of the limits of liability in discussing the various liability coverages. The same basic principle applies to all liability coverages when it comes to the question: "How high should the limits be?" The answer is simple enough: "As high as you can get them." There has been an upward trend in court awards, especially during the last fifteen years, and a home facing a suit with inadequate limits of liability in its policy might well be forced into bankruptcy. The limits for bodily injury should certainly be no lower than $100,000 per person and $300,000 per accident. The limit for property damage should be at least $50,000. In a real sense, the liability exposure is the greatest risk that the home faces, and it should never be neglected for the sake of covering other less important losses.

With the liability exposure covered, we turn to the subject of property insurance. Undoubtedly, the home owns considerable property, including the building, furnishings, perhaps an automobile, and specialized medical equipment. The building probably represents the greatest investment, and this investment should be protected by a fire policy written to cover against fire, extended coverage, and vandalism and malicious mischief. Extended coverage includes protection against the perils of windstorm, hail, smoke, explosion (other than the explosion of a steam boiler) riot, riot attending a strike, civil commotion, and damage done by aircraft and vehicles. If there is a boiler on the premises, it should be covered by a boiler policy. The building should be insured to at least 80 per cent of its value. In most cases of quantity discount, known as the co-insurance rate, the needed insurance can be obtained if the insured agrees to insure the property for 80 per cent of its value. However a word of warning is due here. If the building is insured with a co-insurance provision, the insured obtains the insurance at a lower than normal rate and in return agrees to maintain the specified percentage of insurance to value. If he fails to do so he may be penalized in the event of a loss; this makes it imperative that he review the value of the building periodically to make sure that the amount of insurance complies with the co-insurance requirement.

The contents of the building should be insured against at least the same perils as the building. In addition, there may be some need for dishonesty coverages on the contents. A fidelity bond may be required for those persons who handle the assets of the home. In addition, there may be a need for theft, burglary, and robbery coverage. Perhaps the best policy to cover the dishonesty exposure for a nursing or a retirement home is the Blanket Crime Policy. If written to a limit of $25,000, this single limit contract provides economical protection for fidelity coverage, money and securities on and off premises, counterfeit currency, and depositors' forgery.

Some provision should be made for the exposure of indirect loss which the home faces. The type of policy that will be used to cover the loss of income that results from damage to facilities will depend to a certain degree on the circumstances of operation for each home. If the home will be forced to suspend operations in the event that the facilities are damaged by fire or some other insured peril, the business interruption policy will provide indemnity for expenses which continue while operations are halted. If, on the other hand, the administrator decides to continue operations till the home is rebuilt by moving into temporary quarters (and this may well be the only choice open), the proper policy would be the extra-expense policy. The extra-expense policy would pay the home the amount by which operating expenses exceeded normal. When it is not possible to foretell which course of action would be adopted, it may be necessary to purchase both coverages.

A NOTE ON PACKAGE POLICIES

Insurance is still not a "one policy per customer" business, but the introduction of the Special Multi-Peril program constituted another step in this direction. This program, known as the SMP, is a package policy approach to insurance for commercial risks similar to the homeowners' program in the residential field. The program originally covered motels only, but it has gradually been expanded until it is now possible to purchase a package policy for a wide range of businesses. The portion of the SMP program which is of particular interest to us here is the Special Multi-Peril Institutional Program. Under the provisions and rules of this program it is possible for religious, sanatory, charitable, governmental, or nonprofit organizations to obtain a package policy. Private nursing homes operated for profit are not eligible for the program at the present time.

The aspect of the SMP program that has received by far the greatest attention is the discount which the program provides. Institutional risks such as those listed above are entitled to a 15 per cent discount on the coverages included in the package, and virtually all of the coverages we have discussed may be included. The exceptions are the workmen's compensation insurance and automobile insurance. The package discount makes it possible for the insured to upgrade his insurance program without any additional outlay of premium. There may well be coverages which the administrator would like to have, but which he is reluctant to purchase because of the size of his present premium outlay. The savings realized through packaging his present coverages may permit him to add important coverages (business interruption insurance for example), without any increase in premiums. Administrators who are eligible for a Special Multi-Peril Institutional Program policy should consult their agents.

In addition to those coverages which we have discussed above, numerous other coverages are available. For the most part they are far less important than those that we have discussed. One example is automobile collision. If the budget permits, it may be desirable to purchase this coverage, but it would be unwise to do so at the expense of any of the coverages outlined above. Some of the policies we have not discussed are highly specialized and might be very important for a specific home; each situation is a little different from the others and may require a different approach. The arrangement of a proper insurance program for any given nursing or retirement home is an individual matter and can be properly accomplished only after a study of the property and the exposures that the home faces. However, a little careful study and the right kind of help from your insurance advisor can result in a better insurance program and a better allocation of insurance premium dollars.

The primary function of insurance is in providing protection against losses. The primary rule in purchasing insurance is to make sure that the losses that would be the most damaging financially are covered first. The question the risk manager must ask himself is not "Can we afford this insurance?" but rather "Can we afford not to have this insurance?"

Part Seven

THE ADMINISTRATOR'S PERSONAL AND PROFESSIONAL DEVELOPMENT

Chapter 17

Improving Administrative Effectiveness

WOODROW W. MORRIS, *Ph.D.*

The present-day administrators of nursing and/or retirement homes are, for the most part, self-made men and women. The reason for this is that even a cursory survey across the country reveals that there are practically no training programs designed to develop such administrators. Those which do exist are not only few and far between but also relatively new on the educational scene. However, this will not always be the case.

EDUCATION PROGRAMS PLANNED

With the rapid advances in knowledge and techniques in almost all of the areas of work with which a modern-day nursing home or retirement home administrator must be acquainted, two developments are almost certain to take place. First, it seems quite likely that new formal college training programs will develop, perhaps at the graduate level. They will be designed to train interested students specifically for work in the field of nursing or retirement home administration. It is expected that students with such training will then make this their field of professional endeavor, much as do students now receiving training in hospital and health administration.

The second development will be that of increased activities in extension programs—programs covering all areas with which administrators must be acquainted and in which they work daily. Eventually, these programs will probably reach a level comparable to postgraduate continuing education courses in other professional fields. While the first of these predicted developments will produce professional administrators, the second will help to bring administrators now in the field up to a more nearly professional level of knowledge, competence, and skill. Ideally, such postgraduate courses would become truly "continuation" education courses, keeping both college-trained and "experience-trained" administrators up-to-date with the most recent advances in knowledge.

This, then, brings us to the point of the present discussion of "improving administrative effectiveness" under the conditions as they now exist. Strangely, there are probably more untrained than trained people in administrative positions of all types. Educational programs exist for school administrators and for hospital administrators and a few other types, but even in these fields one finds many persons holding administrative posts who have had little or no specific training. Most of them seem to have "come up through the ranks" or to have learned through experience and trial and error. Thus, while special training may not be essential to success in some cases, it may still be a helpful stimulus to improvement.

In the remainder of this chapter, an effort will be made to touch upon some of the more important aspects of the "good administrator" and how one can strive toward the attainment of this designation.

TRAITS OF THE GOOD ADMINISTRATOR

It may appear to be unnecessary to mention that it is important for the administrator to have a thorough and comprehensive concept of the nature of his calling. Any administrative post which deals with human beings is necessarily complex and exacting; one which focuses on ill or potentially ill human beings is even more so.

Not only is the job demanding, but it is also so broad and so inclusive as to be almost bewildering, including, as it does, such diverse areas as law and tax problems; business procedures; purchasing; general aspects of health; special aspects of diet, nutrition, rehabilitation, mental and emotional problems; recreation; relationships with governmental agencies; and so on.

Whatever the nature of the home or the background of the administrator, there can be no excuse for the neglect of these or any of the other important phases of his job. There can be no excuse, because, in the long view of his work, he is dealing with the welfare of fellow human beings placed, for the moment, in his care.

As an administrator, too, he must remember that he is playing a variety of roles: one for his patients or residents; one for the public at large; one for his fellow administrators, in particular; and another for the personnel on his staff. And, much like the commanding officer of a military base, he should be aware that the morale of his establishment will be fairly directly related to the ways in which he plays these roles. Other things being equal, his roles will be played best if he has a clear philosophy of the nature of his task and of the goals of the institution he heads. What is more, if he is to achieve the breadth of outlook and the depth of understanding which his several roles require, he will need to be an active participant in a wide variety of continuing education programs, provided by local, state, and national professional groups and organizations, including, of course, the American Nursing Home Association and/or the National Association of Non-Profit Homes.

Two special features of the administrator's work stand out: first, the decision-making process; and, second, the leadership role.

Psychologists have given some attention in their researches to an analysis of decision making. Much of this is reviewed in the literature and the reader is referred to the Bibliography for additional readings on this topic. Suffice it to say that decision making depends, in part at least, upon being aware of the main alternatives available; upon making formal or informal estimates of the outcomes of these alternatives; and then, in terms of the problem under consideration, selecting the one or ones most likely to solve the problem and to help achieve the objectives most consonant with the philosophy and goals of the group.

The difficulty in the decision-making process comes in a variety of forms:

1. not seeing the problem itself clearly and concisely
2. lacking awareness of the several significant alternative courses of action
3. maintaining a biased or distorted attitude toward any aspect of either of these
4. being unwilling to accept responsibility for potentially unpleasant solutions or alternatives
5. not seeing clearly the basic goals and objectives of the organization

It is clear, however, that to improve administrative effectiveness in decision making, these difficulties and others like them must be faced, understood, and overcome. This is difficult to do alone; it usually requires an educational approach, the use of skilled consultants, the sharing of problems of this type with professional colleagues, and the sheer gaining of experience in a large variety of decision-making situations.

Leadership is too large a subject to be more than touched upon here and again the reader is referred to the Bibliography for other discussions of this topic. Decision making, of course, is an important aspect of leadership—others probably include planning, policy making, controlling, teaching, directing, and so on. Within the realm of performing these functions in playing the leadership role, one of the most significant and troublesome aspects is not so much "what" is done (as important as that is!) but "how" it is done. The "how" of leadership behavior extends all the way from the autocratic authoritarian speaking *ex cathedra* to the laissez-faire type of leadership (which, incidentally, may well be simply the exercise of no leadership at all). As is true in so many other aspects of life, neither of these extremes is a healthy form of leadership behavior. The former—the autocratic and authoritarian—often only begets grudging, even hostile responses, while the latter begets insecurity, indecisiveness, and, frequently, a chaotic state of affairs.

In the minds of many people there is the belief that some people are "born leaders," or that there are special personality or other psychological characteristics that define the leader. So far, psychological studies of leadership behavior have failed to identify either the former or any isolable traits or personality variables common to known leaders. In a very real sense, this is an encouraging finding, because what it suggests is that leadership is or can be a learned behavior—much like decision making. As such, therefore, improving one's effectiveness as a leader is equivalent to the topic for this chapter, that is, improving administrative effectiveness.

Another aspect of administration comes under the general heading of interpersonal relationships in general, and communications and listening in particular. Much has been written and studied about these topics and the reader is referred especially to two books by Wendell Johnson, particularly his *Your Most Enchanted Listener*.

The effective nursing home administrator must not only be accessible to his staff, to families, to residents, and to those others for whom he plays important roles; he must also be skilled at communicating ideas and feelings, easy and comfortable to talk with, sympathetic and empathic; and, by all odds, a good listener. Over and over again one hears a subordinate, who has been criticized for inept handling of a situation, complain that he *did not understand*. Since the successful administrator depends upon his subordinates for the translation of ideas into actions, it can only be regarded as a failure in leadership if the employee "did not understand." Similarly, in the instance of listening, we tend not to hear people out, to assume that we know what they are going to say, to cut them off prematurely and then behave as though we are following out their thoughts, wishes, or needs.

There is only space here to indicate that communicating and listening can be improved through practice. It does take practice and it usually requires the guidance of experts in the field in order to achieve effective improvement. In a sense this is one of the features of the success of those programs which stress "how to win friends and influence people."

Finally, continuing education is the paramount route to the improvement of all of the various aspects of administration. This is also true of most of life's work. Nowadays, more than ever before, groups at all levels of the occupational scale find continuing education a necessity, if they are to compete successfully for their place in the sun. A recent newspaper headline depicts this graphically: "Farmers Flock to Night School to Keep Up to Date on Agriculture" (Des Moines Sunday Register, February 28, 1965, Page 1, Section F). Another case in point: one whole division of the administration of the University of Iowa College of Medicine is devoted to the devising and administration of postgraduate education programs each year to help satisfy both the need and the demand of physicians to keep up-to-date with the rapid advances of modern medicine. Each year, for example, the College of Medicine plans between fifteen and twenty such courses which are attended by some 1,200 physicians. This is to say nothing of the numerous clinical conferences held under the aegis of various departments of the college. In the 1964–65 academic year, for instance, the departments of Ophthalmology, Otolaryngology and Psychiatry held a total of sixteen clinical conferences—all open to any physicians wishing to attend.

CONTINUING EDUCATION

Both of these examples—and the myriad of others which could be cited—are testimony to the great need for continuing education, advanced education, and just plain education, in order to keep up with the changes taking place in the world today. These changes, as has been noted earlier, apply especially to nursing and retirement home administrators and their staff personnel. The improving of administrative effectiveness in all of its aspects eventually comes down to education as the common denominator. Being cognizant of this fact, the Nursing Homes and Related Facilities Branch, Division of Chronic Diseases, of the United States Public Health Service has a planning committee working on a curriculum (or curricula, if several levels of instruction emerge as desirable) for the training of administrators of long-term care facilities. It is hoped that the course materials thus developed will be widely used by educational institutions, state organizations, and local communities; that eventually the certification of administrators may become an integral part of a nursing and retirement homes licensing code in every state of the Union.

REFERENCES

1. Beal, George M., Bohlen, Joe M., and Raudabaugh, J. Neil, *Leadership and Dynamic Group Action*. Ames, Iowa: Iowa State University Press, 1962.
2. Johnson, Wendell, *People in Quandaries*. New York: Harper & Bros., 1946.
3. ———, *Your Most Enchanted Listener*. New York: Harper & Bros., 1956.
4. Katz, Robert L., *Executive Skills: What Makes a Good Administrator?* Amos Tuck School of Business Administration, June 1954.
5. ———, "Skills of an Effective Administrator." *Harvard Business Review*, January-February 1955.
6. Lee, I. J., *How To Talk With People*. Harper & Bros., New York, 1952.
7. Mace, Myles L., *The Growth and Development of Executives*. Division of Research, Harvard Business School, Boston, 1950.
8. Maier, Norman R. F., *Principles of Human Relations: Applications to Management*. New York: John Wiley & Sons, 1952.
9. Rogers, Carl R. and Roethlisberger, F. J., "Barriers and Gateways to Communication." *Harvard Business Review*, July-August 1952.

Chapter 18

Handling Administrative Problems

LEON I. GINTZIG, *Ph.D.*

An administrative problem is a situation that arises during the normal course of an administrator's day, and requires the making of a decision. Decision making is the selection of a course of action from a group of alternatives. Experience, experimentation, and careful analysis are the bases for decision making.

Therefore, we may define the handling of administrative problems as that which occurs when a manager draws upon his experience and theoretical knowledge (when confronted with a problem), and makes a decisión for solving it consistent with his facilities' policies and procedures.

BACKGROUND FOR MANAGEMENT DECISIONS

There are two important elements in decision making or problem solving, in addition to the factors involved in the actual problem. The first is management policies.

Management policies are basic guides to help the organization reach specific objectives. Sound policies help management handle recurring problems by saving time and making for consistency of action. Three basic types of policies affect the handling of administrative problems: (1) those that are imposed or required by decree (governmental agencies or trade associations); (2) those that are planned by management in advance, in order to guide the actions of those individuals concerned; and (3) those that result from a new problem which might arise from a present policy not being effective.

The second important element in problem solving is that of organization, the type of organizational structure in which you function. For example, if you are delegating responsibilities to others, the problem will be entirely different than if your responsibilities are delegated to you. In the smaller organization, such as the ones with which most of you are affiliated, it is the former rather than the latter situation which will usually exist.

As we will learn later, we must correlate all available facts when handling an administrative problem. Therefore, we should understand what factors are involved in administrative problems. For our purposes we will consider three: human, technical, and economic. Human factors might be those relating to family, health, background ambitions, individual or self needs. Some technical factors might be related to the services offered, the facilities, cost and other financial elements. Some examples of the economic factors are local conditions, market conditions, national and world trends, and the business situations in general.

CHANGING CONCEPTS OF MANAGEMENT

For all organized activity the management function is a most necessary feature. This is true whether the organized activity takes the form of a factory, a bank, a church, a retail store, a hospital, a university, a nursing home, or home for the aged. It is the common denominator which permeates the area of management specialization, such as financial management, ward management, research management, personnel management, and so forth. Moreover, it is a common attribute of the various levels of management in any hierarchical echelon, from the practical nurse group to the top supervisory administrative personnel. As Professor Albers, in his book, *Organized Executive Action,* reminds us, "although the purposes of various organizations differ, the nature of the management function remains constant."

The general management of any business organization as a whole is normally considered to be administration and involves all echelons of management—from the very top down to the supervisory levels. The relationships and performance of the management hierarchy are structured—both organizationally and administratively—to achieve objectives. The traditional managerial functions of planning, organizing, staffing, and so forth are directed toward the attainment of these objectives by the effective use of available resources: equipment, human skills and finances. When administration is using these resources to best advantage, all members of the management team are effectively engaged in the common function of decision making. Recognizing and defining problems, examinining alternative courses of action, and making final choices are stages in the decision-making process. It is the first two phases that require many man-hours of effort; much more management effort is devoted to investigation, fact gathering, and problem-solving analysis in developing courses of action than to the process of selection of the action to be taken. And decision making, considered in this broad manner, constitutes the bulk of managerial activity in regard to problem solving.

The problems that managers at the various levels of the organization face can be classified according to how well structured or how routine they are.

At the lower levels of management are the highly programmed decisions—the ordering of ward supplies, for example. At the higher levels are the unprogrammed decisions—novel and complex problems demanding the skills of the well-trained management person for adequate solution. In fact, there appears to be a rough association between the manager's level in the organization and the extent to which his problem-solving decisions are programmed or not. For example, as the giant corporations have emerged, more and more delegation of managerial responsibility has evolved, and the layering or formation of management steps has occurred.

Today, we tend to think of these levels as top, middle and lower, or supervisory management. And to each has been given a part of the total problem-solving or decision-making process. In addition to these managerial persons, large-scale operations have created opportunities for the staff specialist to participate in the problem-solving function.

In like manner, these various levels of management echelons have developed in the case of the growing health service facilities; but are less evident, at the present time, in the smaller health organization facility.

The first essential of good administration is, admittedly, a sound, professional, managerial attitude on the part of the management employee—a professional interest in finding the best principles and practices of administration, such as the use of the scientific method, what has been called "operations research," and information technology.

Many authorities consider administration an art as well as a science, and these same individuals will use different approaches in solving management problems. In fact, the soundest administrative attitude starts with the proper approach to making decisions. The uses and applications of the various approaches and the results obtained will depend upon the leadership, judgment, and character of the person using them. For while he uses his judgment in making the decisions, he also needs the facts from which to determine those alternative courses of action which, in turn, permit selection of that course of action maximizing the degree of attainment of his desired objective.

PROBLEM-SOLVING TECHNIQUES

Of those methods leading to decision making and determining the solution for administrative problems, I would single out four for particular mention and two will be discussed at some length. The four under consideration are: (1) the scientific method; (2) the administrative function approach; (3) the administrative area approach; and (4) the operations research approach.

THE SCIENTIFIC METHOD APPROACH

This approach has been used to advance our civilization to its high standards of living by enabling its user to solve in the most satisfactory manner the difficult problems which occur. This method involves a clear statement of the problems, the collection of pertinent facts, the analysis and classification of these facts, and the final conclusion based upon these facts.

THE ADMINISTRATIVE FUNCTION APPROACH

This approach is sometimes called the elemental approach and is based upon investigative efforts into the basic and essential elements of administration, such as planning, organizing, coordinating, motivating, and controlling.

THE ADMINISTRATIVE AREA APPROACH

This is based upon certain functions into which a health care organization usually divides its activities, such as medical care, nursing care, engineering service, personnel or human relations department, public and community relations, research and educational services and finance department.

THE OPERATIONS RESEARCH METHOD

This is best described as the application of the scientific method to problems of management, in order to determine optimum solutions.

THE SCIENTIFIC METHOD

In administrative problem solving, the scientific method is first utilized to obtain certain facts. These, in turn, are utilized by the individual administrator, in his own thinking and feeling as he pursues the art of administration. Therefore, it is important that this supervisor use the scientific method in order to obtain more and better facts upon which to base his judgment, imagination, personality, and creativity in the problem-solving process. The basic principle in use here is that all administrative practices are (or can be) caused. In other words, there is a cause-and-effect relationship, and if the administrator finds the cause and changes it, he can change the effect accordingly.

Developments in the management sciences—including statistical decision theory, design of experiments, and operations research (discussed more thoroughly later on)—make it possible to discuss more precisely and more clearly some aspects of the solution of management problems. With the increasing application of management sciences through staff activities, it is most important that administrators understand what information they must furnish the personnel they supervise, if the work performed is to be productive.

What, then, is the administrator's contribution to the application of the scientific approach? I would say that it is to provide, at the minimum, a definite statement of his objectives and goals; an outline of the facilities' policies, resources, and time limitations within which the solutions of the problems are to be sought.

Thus, a preliminary study of a particular situation is desirable to indicate the nature of a problem, its importance, availability of information, availability of techniques to be used, objectives, and resource limitations. These steps are especially useful in establishing communication with decision makers as well as other participants who may have been significant in the effectiveness of the selected solutions. For, despite vast changes in both the tools and techniques of any administrative business operation, one aspect has not yet lost its importance, nor has it been relegated in total to mechanical operation—namely, the human ability to make decisions! I believe it is Walter Finke who, when discussing the area of operations research, implies that for the most part, final administrative decisions will continue to be made by the reliable "Mark I" human being, whether judgment, experience, or intuition is involved.

In selecting this method of attacking administrative problems, I would like to present a framework for the scientific method of approach to problem solutions, consisting of nine individual phases. These will be discussed in such a way as to provide a guide to rational problem solving, in order to achieve objectives.

It should be emphasized here, of course, that although these phases do provide a logical and systematic approach, they do not minimize in the least the need for creativity. Our discussion does cover some conditions which must be met for a thorough investigation and the analysis required in solving a problem. In effect, it is a general framework for solving many types of problems, rather than a specific procedure for a specific problem. The nine phases of problem solving with which we are here concerned are reflected in the following statements:

1. First, determine the problem symptoms by identifying the information and data which lead to a conclusion that improvements should be made or the situation modified.

2. Define the problems by analyzing the symptoms for validity, delineating possible causes of the symptoms, and determining the specific cause or causes.

3. Select a problem by determining the relative significance of the problems, evaluate the costs involved in arriving at a solution, and include the availability of techniques for problem solving, in order to decide which problem, if any, should be approached first.

4. Determine the constraints on the solution by deciding what objectives and goals are to be achieved, what values are to be retained, and what resources are available for solving the problems as an indication of the boundaries within which the solution may be sought.

5. Develop a number of feasible solutions, determine what each one involves, what the possible outcomes are, what is the probability of each outcome, what is its possible use, as well as what is the possible cost of each outcome.

6. Select a solution by applying an appropriate criterion and use it to choose the best of the alternative solutions.

7. Test the solution selected to insure that it will produce the desired result and not an unexpected and undesirable outcome.

8. Plan controls on the solution by setting areas within which the solution will be satisfactory, in order to identify under what circumstances the solution should be considered for change when it is economically justifiable to make a change.

9. Plan a means for implementation of the selected solution, including the details needed for making any modifications necessary to insure its effectiveness.

These nine phases emphasize a problem-oriented approach—that is, making the necessary effort to define significant problems, rather than the solution-oriented approach, which begins by investigating solutions without clarifying the problems. It must be kept in mind, however, that while presented as an ideal process, several practical and economic considerations would determine to what extent the process would be followed.

It should be kept in mind also that the steps common to the formulation of scientific method (the collection of facts, analyzing facts, defining problems, and solving problems) are applicable in every phase of the procedure. And since it is a general process, it is also applicable whether the problems are classified according to the functions of management, the areas of organizational administration, or to some other classification.

The main objective in problem solving is to make the best use of available information, so that the degree of uncertainty is reduced and better decisions are made (analytical procedure).

I have indicated that the first step in the analysis of any problem is to determine the objective being sought. The second step is to decide upon the scope of the problem in terms of variables that can be controlled in its solution. The third step is to develop a method of predicting the extent to which various possible solutions to the problem would accomplish the objective. And the fourth step in the analysis is to find the solution which will best achieve the objective, as determined by the prediction in the third step.

All four of these steps in the analysis are important and frequently difficult; however, predicting the effectiveness of any proposed solution to the problem is the keystone to successful problem solving, since this calls for a theoretical measure of effectiveness of alternative feasible courses of action, rather than determining one by trial and error. It is here, in the third step, that the traditional problem-solving techniques must frequently give way to the newer and more formal operations research techniques.

Although there are many definitions of operations research, it can be defined acceptably in terms of the objectives of management as being a method of providing administrators with a scientific basis for solving problems involving the interaction of all components of the organization, for the best interest of the whole organization. The principal characteristics of operations research may be stated as the use of the scientific method; the use of mixed scientific teams; the systematic approach to problem solving; and the search for optimal decisions to solutions. Let us consider each of these in turn.

First of all, operations research is a prime example of the scientific method. It is, in reality, an organized activity with a more or less definite methodology for attacking new problems and finding definite solutions. Although many management personnel have often used some of the techniques in question, operations research is considered an applied science which utilizes all known scientific techniques as tools in solving a specific problem.

Since most man-machine systems have a physical, biological, psychological and/or an economic and engineering aspect, each of these aspects can best be analyzed and comprehended by a specialist in the appropriate field. But it is generally recognized that no one person's mind can contain all of the potentially useful scientific information, whereas a "team-mind," for all practical purposes, may do so. Consequently, the reasons for the operations research team concept is to bring the most scientific procedures to bear on the problem and to develop new problem-solving procedures as needed. In other words, a mixed-team increases the number of aspects which can be analyzed in detail.

A third factor in this approach is known as the systems approach. The true aim of operations research is to obtain a system or overall approach to problem solving. The term "system" implies an interconnected complex of functionally related components. In fact, it is frequently known as the "holistic" approach, which implies looking at the totality of the operation. The effectiveness of each component of the unit depends upon the way each fits into the whole; and the effectiveness of the whole depends on the way each unit functions.

The final characteristic to be presented is that of the optimum solution. Operations research does not seek merely to find a solution—

or even a better solution—to a problem. Instead, it has as its prime objective that of seeking the optimum solution. However, the final decision to solving the problem rests, of course, with the management person in control of the particular phase of operations. Operations research prepares for action—the team only recommends.

Chapter 19

The Most Difficult Administrative Problems: A Panel Discussion

W. E. KYLE, CHRISTENA NELSON, *R.N.*, and MERTON B. WEINER

A. THE PROBLEM OF ACHIEVING PROFESSIONAL SATISFACTION: W. E. Kyle

Dr. William Moeller of the Psychopathic Hospital in Iowa City, once made an apropos remark when he said that "Nursing homes are expected to be all things to all people." I would add, "Nursing home administrators are expected to be all things to all people." Certainly there are times in each of your daily lives when you would wholeheartedly agree with me. The smaller the home, the more varied the duties one is expected to perform. They may range, actually, from emptying the garbage to dolling up for a presentation to the local Women's Club.

We do live in a busy and complex world; but when people employ our services, they expect us to help them solve what they consider to be a major family or personal problem. Certainly they can expect us to perform these duties diligently in an efficient and business-like manner. This business of providing for and protecting our ill and old is a most serious matter.

I am reminded of a doctor in my home town, who, upon listening to my apologies for calling him in off-duty hours, said to me, "All I have to sell is service." Actually, aren't we in the same position? All we have to sell is service. If we are to be successful in this work, we must continually be reminded (particularly when we might be feeling a little sorry for ourselves) that we entered this service business by our own volition. We knew then that service to human beings was to be demanded of us twenty-four hours each day, every day.

At a recent district meeting of the Iowa Nursing Home Association we heard a most provocative speech by a laywoman whose topic for discussion was "What I See When I Come Into Your Nursing Home." Frankly, she sent me home talking to myself. Her first utterance stopped me. "Why," she asked, "are you a nursing home administrator?" I could think of several reasons why I accepted the job, but only after searching deeply within myself did I know why I am still at the work. Simply put—I am still in this demanding work because it permits me to be of great service to people in great need. This rendering of service to others fulfills a great need within myself. Thus I find myself contented in a profession which is surrounded with human tragedy, pain, suffering, and with death itself. Certainly such surroundings are not conducive to what is normally considered a pleasant setting; but I find my contentment in being of service. Monetary profit alone cannot give me this contentment—nor can lack of profit take it from me.

When I am called upon to render services which at the moment seem "above and beyond," I am really doing that part of my job which satisfies me most. So it is with each of you, I am sure. If it were not, you would not be in the nursing home business.

Your job as an administrator requires great versatility. A primary requirement is knowledge of the field you serve. If I could give you but one key in answer to all your problems, it would be, "Have a thorough and complete knowledge of all you are called upon to do." Under these most favorable circumstances, you would know exactly what to do with every problem; but let's admit that this is an ideal state we cannot hope to achieve.

None of us on this panel claims to have all the answers; but we are representative of a cross section of Iowa nursing homes—the large, the medium and the small, the old and the new. Cumulatively, we represent twenty-five years of experience in the business, and we are here to share the experience of those years with you. Our only certificate in the nursing home business is that of practical experience; but it has been quite an education.

I have stressed service, but only because I feel that we must all be service conscious. If you are, your home will reflect it in your help, your food, your care, your housekeeping, and your public relations.

I would be remiss if I did not present to each of you the services of our own Iowa Nursing Home Association which offers immeasurable opportunity to those in the nursing home field. By meeting regularly with people who have the same everyday problems you do, and by visiting, comparing and listening, you come up with a lot of answers. Association membership is open to all licensed nursing and retirement homes, and your active participation would be another source in your quest for knowledge.

B. THE PROBLEM OF SELECTING, MOTIVATING, AND TRAINING PERSONNEL: Christina Nelson, R. N.

Since the personnel of a nursing home "makes" the home what it is, we are all aware of the vital importance of this phase of our enterprise.

To begin with, we must choose a method of acquiring suitable workers that will reach the section of our population most interested in human service. Newspaper or placard advertising suffices in some areas; television or radio announcements appeal to a different segment. We cannot pass up the possibilities suggested by people we now have in our employ. They certainly would suggest only people with whom they would enjoy being associated; on the other hand, they must be proud of the organization for which they work to invite a friend to come for an interview.

We can eliminate later problems by having an application blank completed on the first interview. An adequate understanding of policy, hours to be worked, time off, vacation periods, and other information is necessary.

The employment agency will also help obtain workers. They should know your wage scales and all other pertinent information in order to be most helpful.

We should not eliminate possible valuable contacts made by callers at the door who seek employment. I particularly like to interview personally any prospctive workers and to do so immediately.

An early physical examination should be required, so as to eliminate people with health problems.

It should be made quite plain to applicants that we seek people with a large degree of patience and diplomacy, because, when trained, they make an invaluable contribution to our organization.

A few days of orientation before beginning training will save wasted time, especially if you have erred in choosing the prospective worker. Let the new prospect work with an experienced employee to expose her gradually to the routine in your home.

Lines of communication must be kept open at all times for personnel to feel at ease. If an administrator is to be away, let it be known where he may be reached and when he can be expected to return.

It is most important for students who are training to be aides to feel that they are expected to be on time for every class and to be responsible for conscientious class work.

Be sure each demonstration is done by every class member, repeatedly, if necessary, to insure her security when she starts "on her own."

Give class members opportunities to ask questions to insure

complete understanding as to conduct, wearing apparel, etc., during the probationary period.

Training without motivation is futile. Job satisfaction comes when cooperation exists between personnel and supervisory or administrative employees.

Many times, trained personnel such as R.N.'s or L.P.N.'s must "unlearn" certain attitudes or procedures in order to fit into the scheme of care in the more relaxed atmosphere of the nursing home.

Placement is another touchy area, because many times friction develops and can only be eliminated when reassignment is tried. Personality clashes must be avoided.

Recognition for excellent service should be rewarded when possible by merit raises. When this is not possible, an expression of appreciation should be made directly to the employee or through the supervisor of the department.

Periodic conferences or round-table discussions can prove very helpful. Enlisting the members of an organization to express ideas relevant to the total effort heightens the self-esteem of individual employees.

C. THE PROBLEM PATIENT: Merton B. Weiner

Most of you are familiar with the term "problem patient." You know that it refers to the patient who presents problems that are not related to the ordinary routine of nursing duties. These problems are sometimes connected with "problem relatives."

The influence of a relative on a patient sometimes results in difficult problems for the nursing staff. The difficulty lies in the fact that the relative is unaware he is doing the wrong thing. This must be pointed out to him as tactfully as possible by the administrator.

How, when, and why should this be done? A good initial step is: Invite the relative into your office for a visit. Arm yourself with all of the facts surrounding the case. These should be available to you from your nursing staff. Know your patient personally so that you will be able to give your own impressions, as well as back up your nurse's statements. Have certain facts before you such as the patient's medicine record, night chart, diet card, diagnosis, and nurse's notes.

When should this be done? When the nursing staff feels that due to the influence of the relative the patient shows a marked change in his behavior. This may mean that his behavior may have changed to being uncooperative or unusually demanding; the resident may show lack of interest in himself and others, or express continuous dissatisfaction with the care, food, and the like.

The question as to why this should be done is the most important. The patient's welfare is at stake, and therefore the reputation of the home. Medication, proper nursing care, and proper diet are all useless if a relative, who does not understand what is being done and why, is constantly upsetting the patient's emotions or attempting to prescribe the medical nursing care themselves.

Let us consider a few of the problems that occur regularly:

1. There is the relative who wants the patient to become an invalid as soon as he is admitted to the home. In this case, the patient is perfectly able to do the most basic things for himself, such as walking, eating, and dressing, but the relative becomes quite annoyed when he finds that we are still allowing the patient to do these things. The relative brought him (or her) to the home so that the nurses could put him to bed, feed him, and dress him. "After all," reasons the relative, "that is what the home is getting paid for."

The administrator should explain that the job of the nursing staff is to encourage the patient to be as active as he can comfortably tolerate; that if we do not let him do as much for himself as possible, he will deteriorate both physically and mentally at an accelerated rate. The relative should be assured that we will not make the patient do things that are not within his physical or mental capabilities.

2. The reverse of this situation is the relative who wants the 95-year-old patient who has suffered a severe stroke to be reborn. This relative continually harasses the doctor and nursing staff to "do something." Often this attitude tends to push the patient beyond his tolerance.

The doctor should be called upon to explain to the relative what he can hope to expect as to the patient's future. The administrator should follow this with an explanation of the nursing procedures that are available at the home and how they will be made use of.

3. There is the patient who tells his relative he is not getting enough food, that the medications are not given properly, that he hasn't had a bath for the three months that he has been here, and so forth. In many such situations the relative believes everything the patient has told him.

The patient, in this case, is likely to have a diagnosis of arteriosclerosis or hardening of the arteries. Its causes, treatment, and results should be thoroughly discussed by the administrator with the relative or relatives. It is sometimes difficult for the relative to understand this problem, and you may find that continuous explanation and reassurance by the doctor, nursing staff, and administrator is necessary.

4. In a special category we would place the do-gooder who would be a friend of the patient. This person usually has nothing better to do every day than to come and visit the patient. He (or she) usually does not confine himself to one patient, but calls on several. The

conversation between this individual and the patient is apt to consist of not very tactful suggestions such as, "My, how terrible you look today"; "It's a shame you have to be here instead of at home"; "Why do your children never come to visit you"; and, "I don't think you are getting the proper medicine."

The do-gooder creates a most annoying problem. It would be well to discuss the situation, point out the difficulties to this person, solicit his cooperation, and try to divert his do-gooder activities into helpful channels. If the person does not cooperate with your suggestions, you may find that stronger measures, such as limiting his visits or even prohibiting him to visit, will be in order.

The guilt feelings of relatives (which are underlying to some extent in all of the cases which I have described) are more often than not the motivating factor in bringing about an unhappy situation. These guilt feelings do not begin when the patient is placed in the nursing home, but have usually been present for a long period prior to this. Many times, complaining or irate relatives are not really unhappy with the home; rather, they are unhappy with themselves. Listen to the complaints and receive them with sympathy. Let the relative "get it out of his system," so to speak, and you will find he will admit how much care the patient was at home. He will probably end up sympathizing with you and apologizing for having burdened you with the patient.

As you can see, it is important that you thoroughly understand the previous relationships between the patient and relative, in order to effectively cope with the present problem. There isn't a family who comes into your nursing home who isn't experiencing an emotional conflict within their family and in themselves. They need your understanding, your patience, and finally, your reassurance. Be ready to offer it to them at every opportunity.

Part Eight

STANDARDS AND REINFORCEMENTS IN THE CARE OF THE ELDERLY

Chapter 20

The Meaning of Accreditation

HENRY A. HOLLE, *M.D.*

The term "nursing home" means many things to the American public. To some it means a glittering, new, streamlined building of modern and attractive design where patients complete their convalescence in comfortable surroundings. To others, it means a dark, crowded, and ill-smelling place where aged people go to die. One wonders if these extremes in the public image of the nursing home are justified by existing conditions.

DEFINITION

The word "accredit" has a somewhat more constant meaning for most of us. It means to be weighed in the balance, if you will, and to be found of high quality. Accreditation has become a sort of status symbol and its value is directly dependent upon the prestige, integrity, and reputation of the accrediting body.

ACCREDITATION INCREASING

Accreditation programs are becoming fashionable in many fields although the process is sometimes called by different names.

In the patient-care field, accreditation of hospitals has been carried on for more than thirty years, first by the American College of Surgeons and later by the Joint Commission for Accreditation of Hospitals. The commission is sponsored by four organizations: The American Medical Association, The American Hospital Association, The American College of Physicians, and The American College of Surgeons. There is strong motivation for hospitals to be accredited because if they are not, they cannot successfully compete for medical interns and residents which are in short supply.

In the United States, our entire system of medical education is based on approved medical schools. Moreover, the American Medical

Association has established an excellent system of medical specialty boards each of which certifies or accredits specialists who have completed the required years of training in approved internships and residences in accredited hospitals. More recently there has been discussion of a need for the accreditation of rehabilitation centers, laboratories, custodial facilities, and the like.

Outside of the field of medicine, we know of the accreditation of schools and colleges and other institutions. Almost everyone seems to want the label of quality and excellence.

NEED FOR ACCREDITATION

In a nationwide inventory in 1961 (*Characteristics of Nursing Homes and Related Facilities,* Public Health Service Publication, #930-F-5, 1963), it was found that approximately 23,000 nonhospital facilities in the United States and territories, with a total of 592,000 beds, provided nursing or supportive services to the aged and chronically ill of all ages. Approximately 11,600 of these facilities were classified as nursing or convalescent homes with 369,300 beds. The other 11,400 facilities with 23,500 beds were classified as homes for the aged, boarding homes for the aged, or rest homes.

In the minds of the general public, however, all these facilities—good, bad, or indifferent—are too often lumped together under the term "nursing home." In view of the great variety of conditions found in these facilities and in the quality of services which they provide, the public image of the nursing home, while steadily improving, still leaves much to be desired. The good facilities suffer along with the bad, and since there has been no nationwide standard under which they could be classified, the poor conditions occasionally brought to light serve to drag down the entire nursing home profession. Even some physicians have looked upon the nursing home as a place to be visited only in case of emergency or to pronounce a patient dead. States have kept the allowable per diem rates for assistance groups to a figure far below that which is required to provide a reasonable standard of care to patients. Thus, a vicious circle has been established. Under a system of uniform assistance payments, facilities which provide a high standard of care are penalized to avoid overpayment of those which provide the lowest standard. Quality of care under such conditions cannot rise to a high level without economic disaster. The need for accreditation thus becomes obvious.

Those who provide insurance coverage for patient care in hospitals are showing considerable interest in the accreditation of nursing homes, because they see opportunities to extend patient coverage to such facilities. However, the insuring agencies have indicated a desire to limit such coverage at this time to facilities which provide "skilled" nursing care by professional or licensed nurses. Again, the need for accreditation is apparent. The general public also expects a higher standard of care in nursing homes than was available in years past. In the short time that the National Council for the Accreditation of Nursing Homes has been in existence, it has received an increasing number of requests for assistance from individuals in their choosing of specific facilities.

The medical profession is also cognizant of a need to distinguish between those facilities which provide good nursing care and those which do not. This was a major factor in the decision of the American Medical Association to join with the ANHA in sponsoring the nationwide accreditation program of the national council.

In view of these considerations the need for accreditation becomes increasingly obvious. Through accreditation it is hoped that the public image of the nursing home in the United States will benefit as has the image of the American hospital over the past thirty years. In the last analysis, however, nursing homes will increase their stature in the same measure as they upgrade the quality of their patient care.

STATE LICENSING

All states now require licensure of nursing homes. In forty-five states Departments of Health are responsible for this program while in five states Departments of Welfare or other agencies are responsible. In the early days of state licensure most licensing agencies concerned themselves principally with such environmental factors as fire hazards and sanitation. A trend toward the addition of regulatory provisions in the field of patient care, including records, is much in evidence. There is also a gradual tightening up of licensing requirements in most states. State licensing agencies also use local agencies whenever feasible to perform inspectional services toward state licensure.

NEED FOR UNIFORMITY

One might raise a question as to why state licensure would not serve the same purpose as accreditation. While licensure has done a great deal to improve the operating conditions in nursing homes throughout the U.S. we are still faced with fifty different sets of laws, rules, and regulations. What is urgently needed is a nationwide uniform standard of accreditation superimposed on a foundation of state licensure. The accreditation program of the national council is designed to meet this need.

PRELUDE TO NCANH

The feasibility of accreditation of nursing homes has been discussed since 1959 between the American Medical Association, the American Hospital Association, and the American Nursing Home Association through a Tripartite Liaison Committee. In May of 1960 the staff of the tripartite committee developed a tentative set of minimum eligibility requirements for accreditation.

During a meeting of this liaison committee in May of 1961, it was suggested that the Joint Commission on Accreditation of Hospitals accept responsibility for administering an accreditation program for nursing homes. The American Nursing Home Association announced that while it endorsed the tripartite committee study plan, it had initiated its own accreditation program.

In August, 1962, the Joint Commission for Accreditation of Hospitals voted to recommend to member organizations that a Division for Accreditation of inpatient care institutions other than hospitals be established within the commission effective January 1, 1963. This division was to be subject to the ultimate and final authority of the joint commission. Apparently, this proposed arrangement was not satisfactory to the nursing home group and ANHA continued its own program of accreditation.

In November 1962, the Board of Trustees of AMA voted that "negotiations be opened with the ANHA with the idea of activating the National Council for Accreditation of Nursing Homes and that the AMA representatives to the Board of Commissioners on the JCAH be instructed to oppose the accreditation of nursing homes by the Joint Commission." As a result of this decision, the JCAH voted in March 1963 "to discontinue any further action toward the development of a program to accredit nursing homes."

ANHA PROGRAM

As previously mentioned, a program of accreditation was initiated within the American Nursing Home Association in 1961. It provided for surveys to be made of facilities applying for accreditation. The reports of these surveys were then reviewed by "state review boards" which transmitted their recommendations to the Central Board in Washington after which certificates were issued or denied. This program was discontinued when the national council established its Chicago office.

ORGANIZATION OF NCANH

The National Council for the Accreditation of Nursing Homes was organized in the spring of 1963. The council consists of two organizational members, namely the American Medical Association and the American Nursing Home Association. The Board of Directors consists of nine members, five physician members being appointed by the American Medical Association and four nursing home members by ANHA. An Executive Director was appointed effective August 1, 1963 and a headquarters office was established in Chicago shortly thereafter.

It should be emphasized that the by-laws of NCANH provide for the admission of additional organization members upon the written approval of member organizations. A recent invitation was extended by the national council to a number of other groups manifesting an interest in the program and willing to participate financially. These discussions are continuing.

DEVELOPMENT OF STANDARDS

Almost immediately, the Board of Directors appointed a Committee on Standards and after several meetings the "Standards for Accreditation" were developed, approved by the board and published. Those who have studied these standards realize that they are quite comprehensive and cover the major items which make up the essentials of a good nursing home. However, they are also quite general in this first edition, and do not spell out detailed requirement under each category.

It was realized that revisions of the standards would be indicated as the program progressed. Because of the urgent need for getting them published and rather widely distributed to those who are interested, such revisions are being deferred for the present. In the meantime, comments and suggestions are invited from those interested in a high quality of patient care.

The decision to accredit at three levels was a difficult one for the Board of Directors to make. Differences of opinion resulted in much discussion and the final decision was to accredit at three levels called intensive, skilled, and intermediate. The difference between them lies in the qualifications of key professional staff.

To be accredited as an Intensive Nursing Care Facility requires the supervision of a registered professional nurse and the presence of a registered professional nurse on duty at all times. In a Skilled Nursing Care Facility, nursing service is under the supervision of a registered professional nurse for a minimum of five days, 40 hours per week. In addition, at least one licensed nurse is on duty at all times. In the Intermediate Care Facility, nursing service is under the supervision of a licensed nurse on duty five days per week with a minimum of 8 hours each day, and a night attendant who is awake and fully dressed.

In general, the standards which govern accreditation are identical for all levels except for these differences in professional staffing. The application is for accreditation only. The level of accreditation is decided by the council after survey of the facility.

The underlying philosophy which prompted the decision to accredit three levels relates to the needs of the individual patient. If a patient's illness is such that a registered professional nurse should be on duty at all times, the attending physician will make sure that his patient is admitted to an Intensive Nursing Care Facility. On the other hand, an ambulatory patient with minimal needs might get along quite well in an Intermediate Care Facility. The rising cost of patient care requires that good judgment be exercised in making the choice according to the needs of the individual patient.

Because of the urgent need to get the national program underway the council is limiting its accreditation to facilities which provide nursing care and therefore it is not accrediting custodial facilities at this time. Should the program be expanded in this direction suitable standards applicable to this group would be developed.

CHICAGO OFFICE

The national council is a nonprofit agency. The budget for 1964 was approximately $200,000. The administrative budget of $100,000 is composed of a contribution by the AMA of $90,000 and by the ANHA of $10,000. A nationwide program such as this is costly and only the expenses of actual survey are paid from survey fees. At the present time the survey fee is $75 plus $1 for each licensed bed.

The Chicago office has a full-time staff of five persons which will be increased as the program expands. A major effort is now being made to recruit able, qualified, full-time surveyors.

I should like to emphasize one point. This is a permanent program. Our office space has been leased for five years initially and all of our office furniture and equipment has been bought outright. We are not a fly-by-night agency.

NCANH PROGRAM

There must be a beginning to all things. When the accreditation program of the national council was established, the Board of Directors voted to give blanket approval to those facilities which had been approved by the ANHA program and certificates of accreditation were mailed to these facilities. Since that time the Chicago office has controlled the processing of all applications, including the appointment of qualified surveyors and their assignment.

After careful consideration, the board voted also to eliminate in processing applications the step which provided for review of individual survey reports by State Review Boards. As applications are received they are first reviewed in the national office and then assigned a surveyor. In addition to the surveyor's report, information is sought from state licensing agencies and other professional sources. The final decision in approving or disapproving an application is made by the Board of Directors of the national council.

As of May 1964, the national council had accredited 287 nursing homes with 18,208 beds. Accreditation has been denied seventeen facilities. Twenty-seven additional applications are ready for survey and many others are in various stages of processing.

The number of new applications being received is very encouraging. The program has received enthusiastic support from the medical profession, including the many state committees on aging. Our goal is not only to recognize high-quality homes through accreditation, but to assist those which are not eligible to improve their standards in order to qualify. For this reason the AMA has encouraged local medical societies and physicians to work with nursing homes in their area in helping them achieve accreditation.

THE SURVEY

An application is not complete until the "Supplemental Information for Surveyor" form has been completed and returned to the Chicago office. The information on this form is carefully checked before a surveyor is assigned to visit the facility. Information in connection with the first ten items, including the state license certificate, need not be mailed but must be available for the surveyor's inspection at the time of the survey.

A specific date for the survey is set when the application is complete and a surveyor is available. A surveyor is then assigned and the facility notified in advance of the survey date, in order to make sure that the administrator and other key staff will be present.

The time required for a survey varies with the size of the facility and the availability of information which needs to be checked by the surveyor. From three to five hours are usually required. An experienced surveyor will notice many things during the survey. In addition to physical plant and equipment, information is obtained regarding the educational background and experience of the administrator; his efforts toward professional advancement for himself and his staff; personnel policies; office management and administrative relationships; adequacy of medical, dental, and nursing care for patients; and the adequacy of the record system.

Restorative measures are of paramount importance, including an underlying philosophy of increasing self-care, activity, and rehabilitation for each patient to the maximum degree possible. Diversional activities to make life in the home pleasant are also looked for. Other essential services are observed including dietary services; medication control; housekeeping; sanitation; and safety measures.

Since good nursing care is the most essential ingredient being evaluated, detailed observations are made regarding the staffing pattern. Patients are also observed for evidence of the quality of care received. The surveyor writes a detailed narrative report upon completing the survey, including a recommendation regarding the eligibility of the facility for accreditation, and suggestions for improving the services observed.

ADDITIONAL SOURCES OF INFORMATION

The national council has additional sources of information which may be of assistance to the board in arriving at a decision. An inquiry is addressed to the state licensing agency as well as to local physicians within the area who have knowledge concerning the facility. These reports are confidential and are used only in processing applications for final action by the Board of Directors.

FURTHER PROCESSING

The staff of the Chicago office, after evaluating all available information, adds its recommendation to that of the surveyor. The board makes the final decision. In accordance with existing by-laws, confidentiality is observed in connection with information in the file of each applicant. As a matter of policy we do not reveal the identity of applicants, unless they have been approved for accreditation. Moreover, every effort is made to assist those who have failed to meet the standards by informing them of their deficiencies. When these have been corrected, they are eligible to reapply for accreditation after a period of at least ninety days.

CERTIFICATE OF ACCREDITATION

If the application is approved for accreditation, the facility and the press are notified as soon as possible and a distinctive certificate is issued in the appropriate level. Each certificate of accreditation bears an expiration date which is usually three years hence, but approval may be granted for only one year under certain circumstances.

Each certificate of accreditation remains the property of the national council and may be revoked at its discretion. Investigation of alleged violations of standards by accredited facilities may be made by the council or its agents at anytime. The decision of the national council with respect to approval of accreditation or revocation thereof is within the sole and absolute discretion of the council.

PROVISIONAL ACCREDITATION

A new facility may not be surveyed before it has completed six months of operation. Provisional approval may then be granted for one year which may be extended to three years without resurvey upon the satisfactory completion of one year of operation. Occasionally, approval is granted provisionally for only one year, pending corrective measures to be taken, in which event resurvey is required.

ACCREDIT ALL GROUPS

There are those who think all nursing homes should be nonprofit; others who think they should be hospital-based; still others who feel that all nursing homes should be controlled by government. This accreditation program is interested in accrediting all qualifying nursing home facilities, whether they be governmental, nonprofit, proprietary or hospital-based. In this connection, I was attracted to a full-page advertisement in the *Wall Street Journal* a few days ago and it went like this:

"IS PROFIT A DIRTY WORD?"

"It's not a dirty word to a little boy or girl who puts a dollar in a bank and expects to get more than that out."

"It's not a dirty word to a newsboy who charges more for his papers than they cost him."

"It's not a dirty word to a widow who puts her and her husband's life savings in blue-chip stocks."

"It's not a dirty word to people who compile dictionaries—who define profit with words like 'good . . . beneficial . . . reward.' "

"Profit is what makes our society go around. By making research and development possible, it makes new products possible . . . and improved products . . . and lower-cost products. It secures jobs and creates new ones. It's essential. It's good."

"Then why do so many businessmen seem ashamed of the word? Why, in annual reports and financial statements and publicity releases, do they hide the word and the idea of profit? Why do they call profit 'earnings' . . . or 'net'? Why don't they call it profit?"

"A banker doesn't apologize for paying 4 per cent interest. Why does a businessman feel the need to apologize when he pays a 4 per cent dividend?"

"We're proud of profit. It's what we're paid to create. It's a good thing to create. It's good, if new products are good . . . if improved products are good . . . if jobs are good . . . if our society is good."

"Let's tell people about profit. They'll understand. It helps them, too."

I need not remind you that the private enterprise system made this country great and that elimination of all profit will not insure economic morality of the highest order. While we in the national council are "without profit" we are reluctant to cast the first stone. We will accredit all types, profit or nonprofit, private or governmental, if they apply and if they meet our standards.

FUTURE OF ACCREDITATION

The effectiveness of this program will depend on several factors. First, it will depend upon the continued high prestige of the national council and the objectivity with which it carries on its program. It will depend upon the availability of a sufficient number of accredited facilities to permit broad coverage on a nationwide basis by large insuring groups. The program depends upon the continued support of the medical profession and of an enlightened discriminating public.

Finally, the effectiveness of accreditation will depend upon the ability of accredited nursing homes to continue their forward progress in improving the quality of their services to their patients.

We would like to see more applications come in from the various states. Many of the older homes are rendering excellent nursing care. Yet we find that quite often they are reluctant to apply for accreditation, because they believe they are not eligible because their buildings are not new. It is believed the administrators of these homes should be encouraged to apply for accreditation if, after studying the standards, they feel that their facilities are providing the quality of services outlined in such standards.

An inspiring story has been handed down from the Napoleonic Wars about a youth who was permitted to carry the regimental banner because he was too young to fight. During one battle, when his unit was advancing under heavy enemy fire, the boy, in his enthusiasm, went so far ahead of the regiment that he was almost out of contact. The regimental commander sent a runner bearing the message, "Bring the standard back to the line." The boy sent back this message: "Bring the line up to the standard." I should like to close my remarks in this vein: Let's bring the homes up to the standards.

Chapter 21

Marshalling Community Resources

H. LEE JACOBS, *Ph.D.*

Homes for the aged in this country have a fairly long history, some having originated more than a century ago. However, the idea of wide community involvement in geriatric care is of comparatively recent origin.[1] Reports from across the country indicate that this socially promising development is less amorphous than formerly; that it is gathering momentum, and is showing evidences of permanency. As persons engaged in promoting the welfare of the elderly, we can be grateful for this turn of events.

The major explanation for this improvement in the breadth of geriatric care is doubtless attributable to such factors as the impact of an aging population, significant advances in medicine, improvements in education and the social sciences, and the proliferation of voluntary organizations. The last of these factors is by no means of least importance.[2]

Until recently, administrators of homes for the elderly put forth little effort to secure help and reinforcement in their work from the community, for two reasons: (1) They lacked understanding of the aging process and the social needs of the aged. (2) They had little faith in the possibility of a worthwhile, sustained response from the community to the plight of the elderly. However, as they have reached out for help, they have often been surprised at the extent and quality of the response which they have encountered.

I recently came upon a story which I think illustrates what is in store for home administrators when they approach their communities with facts and a sincere desire to serve the chronically ill members. In 1754, Horace Walpole, the English writer, in an informal letter to a friend proposed adding a new word to our vocabulary, namely, "serendipity."[3] His proposal was based upon his reading of a fairy tale entitled *The Three Princes of Serendip.* Serendip, as you may recall, was the ancient name for Ceylon. It seems that the princes shared an unusual aptitude. According to Walpole, "As their highnesses traveled they were always making fortunate discoveries, by accident or sagacity, of things which they were not in quest of." Although the term "serendipity" is not often used, it is an intriguing word and is said to designate the happy faculty, or luck, of finding evidence of the correctness of one's ideas, or of coming unexpectedly upon objects or relations which are not being sought. Just as the Old Testament character, Saul, the son of Kish, went forth in search of his father's lost asses, and in his moment of failure encountered the prophet Samuel who informed him that a far greater reward awaited him, namely, the rulership of Israel, even so will the administrator be rewarded, often in ways he does not anticipate, by reaching out to the community in his effort to round out and enrich the geriatric care services of his home.

By "reaching out" I do not mean simply asking for help, though the administrator may profitably and justifiably do this at times, but that he, looking upon himself as a professional person, rather than primarily as a businessman, should participate in all community projects which have as their major objective the improvement of the lot of the elderly. As individuals, groups, and organizations become better informed and motivated, both nursing and retirement homes will be accorded an increasingly vital role in the total geriatric care program. The job that must be done to meet this growing need is obviously too big for such homes to try to handle in isolation. Only an informed and involved community, providing an array of reinforcements for geriatric facilities, will suffice.

What we have said thus far, by way of introduction to our topic, poses three important questions with which we shall be concerned in the remainder of this chapter:

1. Does the administrator have adequate understanding of the ramifications of the geriatric care problem?
2. What is "useful" community activity, as it relates to institutional or congregate living?
3. How can community resources be mobilized and utilized in behalf of elderly patients or guests?

ADEQUATE UNDERSTANDING OF THE GERIATRIC CARE PROBLEM

The principle that "one does well what one understands well" certainly applies to any worthwhile undertaking. Nevertheless, many administrators of nursing and retirement homes are not aware of the magnitude of the geriatric care problem today, as compared to the situation which existed only a generation ago. In 1920, for example, there were only 91,000 persons in this country 85 years of age or older, while in 1960 there were 929,000 in this age category, or an increase of approximately 920 per cent in forty years. Since it is in this age range that the bulk of geriatric care is needed, the rapidly mounting number of "super-oldsters" poses a problem which shows no signs of diminishing in the foreseeable future. In fact, as Dr. Howard A. Rusk, perhaps the most knowledgeable person relative to the rehabilitation potentials of the later years, has pointed out, "The country's general practitioners of medicine are faced with the prospect that 80 per cent of their patients, in a few years, will be people with geriatric disabilities."[4]

OUR CULTURAL UNDERVALUATION OF AGE

In our culture, where the cult of youth and the downgrading of age is still largely the vogue in mass communication, entertainment, social and economic concerns, it is understandable that a great many older persons, especially those among the chronically ill, react in negative fashion to this opprobrious assessment by society; that they so frequently feel "lost" and unjustly used.

While, as we have indicated, the major blame for this dreary picture of old age must be chalked up to the nature of our culture, medical practitioners and their associates of former generations were by no means blameless. Until fairly recently, doctors and nurses were preoccupied with the technical and procedural aspects of treating disease, rather than with treating persons.[5] In fact, they conceived their role—relative to the elderly patient—as being almost exclusively that of easing his pain and of otherwise smoothing his path to extinction. There was an almost total absence of the concept of "rehabilitation"—the "restoration" of "capacities" of oldsters, since they were supposed to have none, at least none worth mentioning.

Around the late twenties, however, some new ideas, sparked by the researches of Thorndike and others, were beginning to invade the premises of education and to "spill over" into related disciplines. These ideas had to do with adult capacities for learning and their persistence beyond age limits heretofore set. Later, social workers and, more recently, medical personnel began to be influenced affirmatively by such views. At first this development consisted mostly of a more favorable picture of middle age. The elderly, though increasing numerically at four times the rate for the general population, were still stranded in the "land of the forgotten."

Then, about a dozen years ago, under the stimulus of important research findings in the field of aging, and by reason of the emerging philosophy of rehabilitation, the plight of the elderly began to be seriously and hopefully considered. Demonstration studies, dealing with the "salvage" of elderly capacities, were initiated and their number increases each year. Already we have learned that rehabilitation rather than mere custodial care of the elderly is a feasible goal; that it pays big dividends—economically, socially and spiritually, even in the case of many geriatric home residents.[6,7,8]

THE NEW DIMENSION OF GERIATRIC CARE

The word "geriatrics" is derived from two Greek words "geras" (old age) and "iatrikos" (healing), and, because our major concern is increasingly with the latter, the whole concept of medical care for the aged is taking on a new dimension of great significance. Says Dr. E. V. Cowdry (often referred to as the "dean among gerontologists), "The treatment of older people represents, in a major sense, a new field of activity. New concepts, new approaches and new services constitute a whole new area of knowledge for the practitioner."[9] The nurse, in particular, has emerged with a much more dynamic and vital role in the care of the geriatric patient than anything known in the past. We might add, however, that these newly created services for the aged and the wider, more hopeful philosophy entailed are by no means in force in all communities.

In thinking more specifically about the needs of the aged, it should be emphasized that there may not be just one, but a number of patterns of good adjustment. For example, some older people seem to thrive on "activity" while others just as ardently prefer quiet and, often, uninterrupted "solitude."[10] Moreover, in the light of what we know about the adjustive abilities of people in all ages, including the elderly, we should sharply reject the assertion of William James, noted philosopher of a former generation, that "the character of the individual is set like plaster by the age of 30 and will never again soften." Individuals of advanced age can and do change and often these changes are in the direction of improvement, rather than of deceleration.

Now that we have cleared the ground and have arrived at affirmative conclusions relative to capacities of the elderly to make adjustments, let us look at some of the adjustmental needs which the aged patient experiences and in the handling of which the geriatric care "team" can and should render an important service. I use the word "should" advisedly since there is now ample evidence to indicate that certain sociological and psychological factors which are an aspect of these needs can cause tension and anxiety in the aged patient, and that these reactions can produce physiological changes in the brain and in the central nervous system.[11] These factors are reflected in what we have come to recognize as "adjustmental needs" of the elderly, especially the geriatric home patient. Though these vary in intensity of expression with different individuals, none can be overlooked without jeopardy to the aged. These needs are:

1. *The need for positive acceptance (e.g., without capitulation*

to hopelessness) of the "fact of aging," including the "losses" which are inevitable with age. The elderly patient needs to understand that "growing older" is a normal and natural process; that "old age" is not a "disease."[12] Such an understanding on the part of the elderly has been found to be positively correlated with good adjustment.[13]

2. *The need for revived self-esteem.* The average aged patient, at least at the beginning of his experience in such a facility as the average nursing home, is apt to suffer from low self-esteem, accompanied by the feeling of rejection, the latter being deeply rooted in the traditional assumption in this country that the older person becomes progressively more worthless to society.

3. *The need to keep open the lines of communication with significant persons, e.g. family members, old friends, and neighbors.* As is to be expected, these relationships tend to be "broken off" in the case of geriatric patients, as families are separated and friends are lost, due to the demands of life and the inroads of death. As studies over the past dozen years have shown, often the very first step in the rehabilitation of the geriatric patient is simply to get him involved in conversation with someone other than himself.

4. *The need for participation in group activity; to belong.* Extreme social isolation is often present in old age, even in homes for the aged or in a hospital ward. While we do not know for sure what makes for a "good life" in old age, we believe, with Dr. Leo Simmons, that the "key" may well be "social participation"—to the very end, if possible.[14]

5. *The need for social recognition and acceptance.* The famous "four wishes," first annunciated a generation ago by the sociologist, W. I. Thomas, apply not only to youth, but to all other ages as well. They are:

(1) the wish for Security
(2) the wish for Recognition
(3) the wish for Response, and
(4) the wish for New Experience

Contrary to popular opinion, the wish for *security* does not necessarily take precedence over the other three, so far as the aged are concerned. In fact, most aged patients would rate *recognition* and *response,* which imply acceptance and esteem by significant persons, as their deepest need. They would agree with the ancient sage who said, "Better a crust of bread where love is, than the security of riches."[15]

6. *The need for renewed confidence in his capacity for improvement; for a sense of "on-goingness."* The average elderly patient, sharing a widely held opinion, is convinced that his mental powers have certainly "faded"; that a nursing home is the "end of the road," the "place where one goes to die." Such patients need repeated re-

assurance by the administrator, the nurse and her colleagues that, as Cicero pointed out two thousand years ago, "the old retain their intellectual powers, provided their *interest* and *inclination* continue.[16]

7. *The need for a more positive "image of aging."* The aged, no less than the general public, tend to succumb to "old wives tales" relative to the meaning of "old" in our society. Traditionally, "old age" has been equated unequivocally with loss and with both mental and physical deterioration, thus leaving no room for the possible assets of later years. An important part of the *improved image* which is needed must begin in the attitude of the administrator and his staff.

8. *The need to gain and maintain status—a position as a significant person in his own world, however defined.* There is no substitute for a vital function at any age, even among the elderly.[17]

9. *The need for "future orientation"—a hopeful outlook on life; a realistic optimism.* Some reminiscing is normal, even beneficial, but excessive dwelling in the past, a shortcoming shared by most geriatric patients can defeat, if not halted, all attempts at restoration. This can best be accomplished by making sure that the "conditions of living" in the geriatric home are warm, inviting, and stimulating.

10. *The need for religious participation, primarily because it supplies contact with the "fellowship of those who care."* Concern of the elderly patient about such matters as bereavement, loss of a sense of worth, and death, calls for answers which religion, through the instrumentality of the church, can give most convincingly.[18,19]

USEFUL COMMUNITY ACTIVITY, AS IT RELATES TO INSTITUTIONAL OR CONGREGATE LIVING

A useful community activity, institutional or congregate, as it may be related to geriatric living, may be defined as any activity provided by the community which contributes to the effectiveness of the nursing and/or retirement home in its objective of helping the patient or guest meet his adjustmental needs, thereby attaining what one geriatrician refers to as "maximum self-sufficiency and independence in a reasonable time and at a reasonable cost."[20] To the considerable number of administrators of homes for the aged who still regard chronic illness as "inherent" in aging and therefore irreversible, this rehabilitative point of view makes little sense.

As recently as 1959 an official government report indicated that very few nursing homes provided casework service, and not many provided activity programs of any kind for elderly patients.[21] This, despite the fact that recent studies have shown that the lack of social participation in old age is more important than "age," as such, as a factor in "social withdrawal" and subsequent mental and physical decline.

POTENTIALS FOR PATIENT RESTORATION

This knowledge calls for a radical change in our approach to the care of the half million aged confined to hospitals and nursing homes, as well as to perhaps an even larger number of noninstitutionalized elderly who receive a lesser level of geriatric care. Chronic illness and disability are not inevitable consequences of aging, but about 40 per cent of all chronic disability is accounted for by persons 65 years of age and over. However, when such afflictions do occur, they are usually amenable to treatment. And no small part of that treatment is a comprehensive rehabilitation program, which includes the utilization of a wide range of community resources. A report by the Illinois Public Aid Commission on a 1956 study-demonstration project is a case in point. That project, which involved thirty-six nursing homes throughout the state, showed conclusively that an effective rehabilitation program at the nursing home level is a feasible undertaking for a home of any size. What is more, this project has shown that even in cases where the program has not resulted in the return of some patients to their own homes, such patients have willingly accepted the responsibility for increasing their own self-care.[22]

The growing recognition of the dynamic nature of illness and the potentials in the human organism for restoration of function has brought into being a greater variety and flexibility in institutional programs for elderly patients. In fact, recent demonstrations in several states, including New York, Pennsylvania, Michigan, Illinois, and Iowa, indicate that up to 50 per cent of present nursing home patients, if given opportunity for exposure to a comprehensive rehabilitation program, would no longer require institutional care—that is, provided independent housing, foster home care, and continued supportive social (community) resources were available. These latter include such state services as those supplied by the Family Service Agency, rehabilitation centers, community centers, Golden Age clubs, the Public Welfare Department, the Community Committee (or Council) on Aging, chronic illnesses information center, geriatric screening clinic, the Friendly Visitors organization, church groups, and many other voluntary associations. Not all of these will be found in every community, to be sure, since every community is unique, but no American community is without some helpful resources upon which administrators of homes for the aged may call.[23,24,25]

VOLUNTEER HELP AVAILABLE

It is estimated that more than thirty-five million persons in the United States are engaged in volunteer work of all kinds.[26] Volunteer effort is basic to our American way of life and it is one of the reassuring and distinctive parts of our democratic thinking and action.

While, to be sure, not all of these millions of people are available for assistance with geriatric patients, the number of persons who are willing and eager to "lend a hand" in work with older people, both the sick and the well, is growing steadily.

The great healing and restorative value of planned activity within a social framework is at long last beginning to be understood. This therapeutic use of the social and cultural environment represents a "stretching" of the concept of what is known in hospitals as the "therapeutic community." The term originally had reference to a new teamwork approach to treatment of mental disorders in a psychopathic hospital.[27] More recently it has had limited application in some general hospitals, and there is a growing awareness of its importance in the nursing home field. This notion of the "total" therapeutic community calls for more coordination of activities than ever before. Beautiful buildings and grounds, expensive equipment, and an efficient staff are not enough. To these must be linked a network of community services, tapped continuously with imagination and skill.

HOW COMMUNITY RESOURCES CAN BE MOBILIZED AND USED

The first step in the use of community resources in behalf of the geriatric patient should be a thorough investigation of the patient himself—what he does or has done in former years, what his potentialities, interests and hobbies are, or have been.[28] This often affords valuable clues to the patient's former community connections which can be used for his continuing benefit. Quite frequently, also, the administrator will discover that certain patients share some community interests and that they will profit greatly by being brought together, even though in wheelchairs or, as in some cases, "flat on their backs."

The point which I wish to make here is that many patients, with a little understanding assistance from the administrator, nurse, and others in charge, can easily learn to help and strengthen one another. What is more, it has been my observation, based on extensive contacts in general hospitals, nursing homes, and retirement homes, that many patients derive deep satisfaction from such activity. At the same time they receive healing and restorative values which they are not likely to derive in any other way. For example, in Boston there is an organization known as Q.T., Inc., the members of which are exclusively persons who have undergone ileostomy surgery. This group provides visitors for ileostomy patients, prior to surgery. The latter can then "identify" psychologically with these Q.T. members and be helped by them in their adjustmental problems during the remainder of their stay in the hospital, and after they have returned to the community. Here we see the "medical team" reaching out to the community in its effort to help meet the adjustmental needs of patients of various age levels, including the elderly.

MOTIVATION THROUGH ACTIVATION

Unfortunately, however, as Dr. Esther Brown points out, "Medical and nursing staffs have had little orientation toward, or preparation in, finding out about patients' social backgrounds, interests, and desires as a basis for considering how these can be used for therapeutic purposes." The physiologically based attitude toward patient care continues to be the major frame of reference in many places. The idea of "patients aiding other patients" and of using adult patients as "team members" and consultants in general hospitals, to say nothing of nursing and retirement homes, is still fairly "strange talk" to many members of the healing art. They are not yet convinced that time spent in observing, interviewing, listening to, and motivating elderly patients is justified; nor that it should be classed under "nursing procedures," which have traditionally cast the patient in the role of recipient and never the giver.

In the average American community there are a great many resources outside the geriatric home or the hospital upon which the administrator and his colleagues may call for vital assistance in meeting some or all of the ten major adjustmental needs of elderly patients previously discussed. Enlarging upon the list of resources mentioned earlier, I would include families of the patients; individual churches, which may be broken down into individual members, groups, organizations, and clergy; the Social Action Committee of the Council of Churches; the local branch of the Family Service Association; the Community Committee or Council on Aging, Senior Citizens Center, groups or clubs; local branches of the Federated Women's Clubs, every one of which, in Iowa at least, has a committee on gerontology; service clubs, most of which now have a special committee on "senior citizens" or "service to the aged" which, in turn, is affiliated with a national committee; the Public Welfare Department; the public library, representatives of which are happy to make regular "rounds" in geriatric homes, when invited to do so; Gray Ladies, Voluntary Workers' Council, and Friendly Visitors groups, the members of which have at least had some informal training in visiting the elderly, including those who are in homes for the aged.

In one small community, Earlham, Iowa, the administrator of a new nursing home facility has, at the invitation of a local committee, assumed the leadership of a well-known home care program. With the help of his wife as assistant administrator, his objective is now to help elderly persons to remain interested and involved in the affairs of life, whether in their own homes or as patients in his nursing home. This is probably the only arrangement of its kind in the nation and will doubtless be watched with a great deal of interest by leaders in the field of geriatric care.

One of the most outstanding examples of successful utilization of community resources in the care of geriatric patients which has come to our attention is to be seen in the policy which has been espoused in all Wisconsin county homes for more than twelve years. That state now has a full-time "director of activities" for its county homes, who works with the staff in each institution on the job of keeping residents functional and participating in activities which are stimulating and personally rewarding. Judging from reports in their bimonthly publication, *The Oldster,* every helpful aspect of community life surrounding these homes is "tapped" in behalf of the elderly residents and with dramatic results.[29] In our opinion, Wisconsin is unexcelled in the imagination and thoroughness with which it deals with perhaps the most needy segment of its population. And, we might add, what can be done in a "county home" can certainly be accomplished in the average nursing or retirement home.

Motivation of the elderly to keep physically alert and mentally active often stems from very simple procedures within their own ranks, rather than from the fanfare of elaborate community plans in their behalf. For example, in one small Iowa county seat town a retired chemist, with a deep interest in reading and public affairs, decided to try to help the older men of his community, most of whom seemed to be drifting into a state of physical and mental lethargy. Accordingly he sent out a personal invitation to several old friends, addressing them as "Fellow Senior Citizens" and inviting them to join him in a meeting in the basement of the public library "for the purpose of fellowship and the consideration of mutual needs."

At the first meeting nine men, ranging in age from 65 to 87 years, and in former occupations from farmer to county school superintendent, were in attendance. Out of their deliberations on that occasion came the decision to adopt a project entitled, "Let's Promote the Library." Within two months the librarian reported a 20 per cent increase in book withdrawals.

The search for new activities led this group, eventually numbering 25, to inquire about needs of the elderly in their community. From the information thus obtained they drew up a list of "needs" for the purposes of group discussion and possible action. Many community problems, as they related to the elderly, were brought under scrutiny and several were acted upon. Some of the literature, including a selected number of books on aging, collected for the weekly discussions, eventually became a section in the local library. Besides participating in the regular meetings of the group the members visited incapacitated older friends in the hospital, nursing homes, and private homes.

For residents of nursing and retirement homes who have experienced major visual loss, an excellent motivating experience can be provided through the use of "talking books," which may be obtained free from the Commission for the Blind located at the state capital in most states. A wide variety of literary materials are available, including recordings of the *Reader's Digest* and major books of the Bible.

Other types of activation which may be realized with some nursing home patients and certainly with many retirement home residents, include instruction in such matters as bridge, chess, lipreading, and typing. In several communities, such activity has been made available through the adult education division of the public school, with instruction sessions being conducted within the nursing or retirement home itself. In one retirement home the typing and lipreading classes each enrolled approximately twenty residents, with splendid results from the standpoint of the participants. In the same home, instruction in the game of chess was provided by a retired dentist.

REINFORCEMENT FROM A "CITIZENS BOARD"

Another more widely based approach to the mobilization and utilization of community resources in the interest of all types of geriatric care is to be seen in another midwestern state, Indiana. There a concerted effort is being made to enact legislation requiring county homes and public homes to establish a "citizens board." Several of the proprietary and nonprofit homes in that state have already set up such a board and are reported to be well pleased with the arrangement. They have found that these citizens groups provide excellent "sounding boards" for any home; a means of objective interpretation of policies and activities to the rest of the community. In addition, they provide a source of expert knowledge upon which the administrator can feel free to call in the improvement of his day-to-day operations.[30]

The "citizens board" should be as representative as possible, including people from business and industry, politics, medicine, welfare, farming (in small communities), "senior citizens" clubs, churches, recreation departments, service clubs, public libraries, adult education classes, and other categories appropriate to the particular community. With this type of group as both a "sounding board" and reinforcement for the home, its needs and those of its patients or guests are apt to receive more serious consideration than they otherwise would. The modern nursing and/or retirement home can no longer be conceived as a "one-man," one-church, or one-organization project. Neither are residents of these homes to be looked upon as "aliens" in the community; they must be made to feel they are a part of it. Community involvement in carrying out the program and purposes of the home, of whatever kind, is, therefore, paramount. Only in this way can the wide range of resources available in most communities—health, medical, educational, legal, economic, recreational, and social—be adequately utilized.

EXPERIMENTS IN PUBLIC RELATIONS

Many methods for creative handling of public relations in a nursing and/or retirement home have been experimented with. For obvious reasons, of course, the public relations problems of nursing homes are ordinarily more acute and exhibit wider ramifications.

Among the more difficult problems faced by most nursing home administrators are those associated with the patient's own family, relatives, and/or other supposedly well-meaning "visitors." In the case of the family, however, it should be said that, contrary to widely held opinion, most elderly nursing home patients are not simply "dumped" or "put away" in such an institution by "heartless middle-aged children," or other relatives.[31] In many instances, there exists a deep, corroding sense of guilt on the part of the adult children involved, and, almost invariably, there are ambivalent feelings which come into sharper focus at such a time.[32] This situation calls for sympathetic understanding and imaginative handling, rather than wholesale condemnation. In many cases, the taking of an aged parent or other relative to a nursing home, or other geriatric facility, is the best and most humane solution to a family problem. But the final decision to do so is seldom easy.[33]

One nursing home administrator, who is also a registered nurse, follows what I consider to be an admirable approach to the utilization of the family in behalf of her elderly patients.[34] When some member of a prospective patient's family makes inquiry, this nurse-administrator spends considerable time in "finding out all the facts about the elderly person's background, interests, and needs." Prior to his (or her) entrance into the nursing home, she goes for several visits with the family and the elderly member in particular. Together they try to reach some common ground of understanding about all that will be involved, and the adjustments that will need to be made on the part of all concerned. Then, on the day the new guest comes to the home to live, this small home administrator has extra help available. In this way, she can give "undivided attention" to the new resident and thus become better acquainted with his (or her) wants, likes, dislikes, and ailments, both mental and physical. She subsequently works quite closely with the patient and the immediate family, in meeting adjustmental problems as they arise. She encourages the family to confer with her frequently, to offer criticism and to make suggestions, relevant to the improvement of her program at any time. Her aim is to make her nursing home a "true home," rather than a "vegetation center." In order to do this she says, "I must encourage all kinds of therapy." Among these therapeutic resources, she considers the patient's family by no means of the least importance. While admittedly such a procedure might not be considered feasible for a large home, the principle involved is universally valid.

VISITORS—PROBLEM OR OPPORTUNITY?

One of the most universally perplexing problems in nursing homes seems to be that of dealing with "visitors" of all degrees of consanguinity or none. Many ways have been hit upon for dealing with this problem. In some cases the results have been so satisfactory that visitors have, in the main, been listed as "assets," rather than "liabilities," in the running of a home. In one large nursing home, the administrator has, for several years, followed the policy of holding occasional informal sessions with relatives and other home visitors, at which times many problems are "aired," questions answered, and information given out as to home procedures. This has reduced adverse criticisms of the home virtually to the vanishing point.

In another community the administrator of a sixty-bed home has found that an occasional picnic or outing to which both patients and family members are invited provides ideal opportunities for clearing up misunderstandings, promoting goodwill for the home, and, not of least importance, providing therapeutic values for patients.

Other goodwill building measures that have been tried with gratifying results include:

1. visitor's suggestion box
2. handout folder on home policies
3. women's auxiliary for procuring and training volunteer workers
4. open house on many anniversary occasions
5. public school children's chorus and other community music groups entertained on festive occasions, in spring and fall, on nursing home grounds
6. conducting a nurses' aide course at the home, to which all interested persons are invited. In one eighty-bed home in an Iowa town of 1,300 population, where this has been tried, the administrator reports a waiting list of women who wish to take this course because they expect to use the information in their own families, rather than as job training. Needless to say, here is one device for brightening the "public image" of any home. This particular home has enjoyed 100 per cent occupancy since the end of its first year, despite widespread gloomy predictions from townspeople and others prior to opening.

CLERGY AND CHURCH GROUPS AS A BASIC RESOURCE

A community resource that is almost universally available in the care of the geriatric home patient is the church, with its varied leadership and organizational ramifications. Several studies have shown that religion, especially as expressed in church attendance and in participation in church activities, is significantly related to various indicators of the personal adjustment of older people.[35]

Ordinarily the first step in the use of this important resource is contact with the clergy. Frequently, a family desiring information relative to a suitable nursing home or other type of geriatric facility as well as guidance in dealing with an aged member, will call first upon their minister, priest, or rabbi. In any case, if he has had adequate professional training, he, more than any other person outside the family circle, except possibly the family physician, is likely to have helpful influence with the elderly patient. His help and counsel should be sought from the beginning.

Other important help from the church is often supplied by the laity, functioning through organizations and committees. For example, in one Iowa church a special visitation committee, made up of middle-aged and older women who had considerable leisure time and ample means, averaged 500 "calls" per year for several years on elderly shut-ins in geriatric homes, hospitals, and private homes. They "remembered" the aged patients on birthdays and holidays with special greetings and other tokens of friendship and affection. They also arranged for "recordings" of church services and special occasions to be used in calls upon shut-ins of all ages, including aged patients. Some of these older people especially enjoyed having these "friendly visitors" read to them, while others preferred a chance to talk to someone who, they felt, would listen sympathetically and understandingly. Comments made by many of these oldsters indicated that such friendly visits and other manifestations of goodwill by church people meant more to them than anything else that had been planned for them.

In some communities the local Council of Churches, in cooperation with other interested groups, is able to bring about a more effective focusing of community resources for helping to meet the adjustmental needs of elderly patients. The nursing and/or retirement home administrator should not hesitate to call upon any of these resources. However, as we indicated earlier in this chapter, he should first of all be an active supporter of and worker in community activities himself.

HANDLING RECENT LEGISLATIVE PROVISIONS IN THE INTEREST OF ELDERLY PATIENTS OR GUESTS

Two pieces of legislation signed into law on July 14 and 30 of 1965 respectively—the Older Americans Act of 1965 (H.R. 3708), and the Social Security Amendments of 1965 (H.R. 6675, popularly known as "medicare")—call for continuing scrutiny by administrators.

These provisions for the elderly are, in the words of President Johnson, "aimed at meeting the needs of our older citizens at the home town level." The health bill (H.R. 6675), in particular, will entail maximum utilization of nursing homes, and, to a lesser extent, retirement homes. Administrators of both types of facilities must be ready to meet the requirements of this unparalleled advance in health care of the elderly.

Among the "musts" for nursing homes, in particular, if they expect to take full advantage of the "medicare" program, will be: accreditation (or its equivalent); a working agreement with a hospital or hospitals; a utilization review; a supervising registered nurse, with licensed nurses around the clock; and submission of cost figures to establish payment for services. These requirements will result in extensive changes for many nursing homes. However, with the expert guidance from state and national association officials and leaders which is now available, cooperating local home administrators will find the task of adjustment to the new program much less arduous than many have anticipated. What is more, they can move ahead with confidence that nursing homes will be looked upon, without question, as vital members of the community health care "team"; and that more adequate payments will be forthcoming for such quality services rendered.

In order to become well informed on these important matters, nursing home administrators who have not already done so should obtain from the Social Security Administration two booklets on the new health insurance and medical insurance programs for the aged, titled, "Social Security Amendments of 1965," and "Health Insurance for the Aged." The first of these contains information for those who provide services authorized under the new Social Security Amendments. The second booklet is a question-and-answer discussion of requirements.

While the Older Americans Act of 1965 (H.R. 3708), which became law less than one month before the enactment of H.R. 6675, has an important bearing on the health of the elderly, it is aimed primarily at the concerns of the well, older population.

The three chief provisions of the bill are:

1. Establishment within the Department of Health, Education and Welfare of an Administration on Aging; a Commissioner on Aging appointed by the President and confirmed by the Senate; and the setting up of an Advisory Committee on Older Americans. The director of this new Administration is William D. Bechill, Commissioner of Aging. It is hoped by the sponsors and supporters of H.R. 3708 that the many federal programs affecting older people which

have been parceled out to many departments and agencies can now be enhanced by being brought together under the new Administration on Aging, and thereby extricated from the "welfare approach" which is resented so bitterly by many proud and independent older Americans.

2. Provision of grants for community planning, service, and training for the development of new or improved programs for older citizens. These grants, totaling $5,000,000 for the first fiscal year and greater amounts in subsequent years, will be allocated to the states, to be administered by Commissions on Aging or other agencies responsible for senior citizens' programs.

3. Provision of grants for research, development, and training projects. These grants will be made to public or nonprofit private agencies, organizations, or institutions, the purpose being to stimulate the study of patterns and conditions of living of older adults and to discover ways for making their lives more wholesome and meaningful. This will include the development of new approaches, techniques, and methods. In addition, specialized training of persons employed or preparing for employment in carrying out programs related to H.R. 3708 will be financed by these grants.

Since the main work of administrators of retirement homes, in contrast to that of administrators of nursing homes is with well older persons, it would be advisable for them to look into the provisions of the Older Americans Act and to take advantage of the varied resources it affords.

CONCLUSION

The community must assume greater responsibility toward the aged, not only for the sake of the well-being of the latter, but because of its own as well. The generally held pessimistic viewpoint, relative to rehabilitative possibilities in the care of geriatric patents, is unjustified. We should be able, with the help of an informed and motivated citizenry, to do for and with our elderly, including the physically ill and emotionally disturbed older patients, as much as we are now doing for the child, which, I think all must agree, is considerable.

FOOTNOTES

1. Zelditch, Morris, "The Home for the Aged—A Community." *The Gerontologist,* 2:1:37–41, March 1962.
2. Rose, Arnold M., Ph.D., "The Impact of Aging on Voluntary Associations." *Handbook of Social Gerontology: Societal Aspects of Aging.* Tibbitts, Clark (ed.). Chicago: University of Chicago Press, 1960, pp. 666–97.
3. Rapport, Samuel and Wright, Helen (eds.), *Great Adventures in Medicine.* New York: The Dial Press, 1961, pp. 516 ff.
4. Rusk, Howard A., M.D., "Rehabilitation—An Economic and Social Necessity." *Rehabilitation Record,* 2:2:19–20, March-April 1961.

5. Brown, Esther L., Ph.D., *Newer Dimensions of Patient Care: The Use of the Physical Environment of the General Hospital for Therapeutic Purposes.* New York: Russell Sage Foundation, 1961.
6. Donahue, Wilma, Ph.D., "An Experiment in the Restoration and Preservation of Personality in the Aged." *Planning the Older Years,* Donahue, W. and Tibbitts, C. (eds.). Ann Arbor: University of Michigan Press, 1950, pp. 169 ff.
7. ———, "Research on First Admission Geriatric State Mental Hospital Patients." *Age, Disability and Rehabilitation.* Proceedings of the Second Annual Conference of the Iowa Rehabilitation Association, October 22, 1963, The Institute of Gerontology, University of Iowa.
8. Masterman, L. E., "Some Psychological Aspects of Rehabilitation." *Journal of Rehabilitation,* 24:4: 4–6; 26, July-August 1958.
9. Cowdry, E. V., Ph.D. (ed.), "The Care of the Geriatric Patient." *Community Organization and Programs.* St. Louis: C. V. Mosby, 1958, pp. 372–90.
10. Kuhlen, Raymond G., Ph.D., "Aging and Life Adjustment." *Handbook of Aging and the Individual: Psychological and Biological Aspects,* Birren, J. E., Ph.D. (ed.) Chicago: University of Chicago Press, 1959, pp. 852–97.
11. Wolff, Kurt, M.D., *The Biological, Sociological and Psychological Aspects of Aging.* Springfield, Illinois: Charles C Thomas, 1959.
12. Weller, C. V., M.D., "Biologic Aspects of the Aging Process." *Living Through the Years,* Tibbits, C. (ed.), 1960, p. 27.
13. Williams, Richard H., Ph.D., "Changing Status, Roles and Relationships." *Handbook of Social Gerontology: Societal Aspects of Aging,* Tibbitts, C. (ed.), 1960, pp. 261–97.
14. MacRae, R. H. (ed.), "The Individual and the Community." *Background Paper on Local Community Organization.* White House Conference on Aging, January 9–12, 1961, pp. 6–11.
15. Proverbs 17:1 (RSV).
16. Cicero, *De Senectute* ("Concerning Old Age"). *Aging in the Modern World,* Tibbitts and Donahue (eds.). Ann Arbor: University of Michigan Press, 1957, pp. 118–33.
17. Burgess, E. W., Ph.D., "The Growing Problem of Aging." *Living Through the Years,* Tibbitts, C. (ed.). Ann Arbor: University of Michigan Press, 1951, p. 12.
18. Gray, R. M., Ph.D. and Moberg, David O., Ph.D., *The Church and the Older Person.* Grand Rapids: Wm. B. Eerdmans, 1962, pp. 39 ff; 126; 130; 134 ff; 142–47.
19. Jacobs, H. Lee, Ph.D., "Spiritual Resources for the Aged in Facing the Problem of Death." *Adding Life to Years,* Bulletin, Institute of Gerontology, 6:3:3–8, March 1959, University of Iowa.
20. Chapin, Sidney, E., M.D., "Home Care for the Chronically Ill Geriatric Patient." *Journal of the Michigan State Medical Society,* 58:9:1463, September 1959.
21. U.S. Senate Report, *The Aging and the Aged in the United States,* 1960, p. 139.
22. Larson, Leonard W., M.D. (ed.). "Community Health Programs for the Aging." *Background Paper on Health and Medical Care,* White House Conference on Aging, January 9–12, 1961, pp. 38–71.
23. Hale, Mark, Ph.D., "Community Services for Aging Citizens." *Counseling the Older Disabled Worker,* Muthard, J., Ph.D. and Morris, W. W., Ph.D. (eds.), pp. 93–98.
24. Harris, Opal, R.N., *A County Health Department Geriatric Program.*

Case Study No. 9. U.S. Department of Health, Education and Welfare, Washington 25, D.C., 1961. Price, 15¢.

25. Byron, Evelyn S., *A Friendly Visiting Program.* Case Study No. 13. U.S. Department of Health, Education and Welfare, Washintgon 25, D.C., June 1961.
26. Allan, W. Scott, *Rehabilitation: A Community Challenge,* especially Chapter 19, "The Community Responsibility." New York: Wiley & Sons, 1958, pp. 172–79.
27. Patterson, C. H., *Counseling the Emotionally Disturbed.* New York: Harper & Bros., 1958, pp. 124 ff.
28. Thompson, P. W., M.D., "Let's Take a Good Look at the Aging." *American Journal of Nursing,* 61:76–79, March 1961.
29. *The Oldster: Newsletter for the Wisconsin County Homes.* Madison, Wisconsin, 9:2:32, March-April 1962.
30. Breen, Leonard Z., Ph.D., "Community Resources for the Rehabilitation of the Older Client." *Counseling the Older Disabled Worker.* Muthard, J. E. and Morris, W. W. (eds.), pp. 85–92.
31. Arth, M., West, J., Blau, D., Kettell, M., "Family Disinterest as a Factor in the Mental Hospitalization of the Aged." Unpublished Report, Geriatric Hospitalization Project (Boston), 1962.
32. Anonymous, "We Sent Mother to a Nursing Home." In *Saturday Evening Post,* June 1956.
33. Spaulding, J. C., "Nursing Homes." *Today's Health,* February 1955, pp. 46 ff.
34. Rogers, Esther, R.N., "Personal Adjustment to the Nursing Home." *Adding Life to Years,* Bulletin, Institute of Gerontology, University of Iowa, October 1959.
35. Cavan, R. S. *et al., Personal Adjustment in Old Age.* Chicago: Science Research Association, 1949.

Chapter 22

The Role of the State Department of Health

FELIX W. PICKWORTH, *B.S.* and WALTER W. LANE, *B.S.*

The role of the State Department of Health in relation to nursing homes and other types of long-term care facilities varies somewhat in the different states. For example, all states now have licensing requirements, but in five (New York, Rhode Island, New Jersey, Louisiana, and the District of Columbia) the licensing is done by agencies other than the State Health Department.

In Iowa, the State Department of Health has been designated by the state legislature as the licensing agent for nursing and custodial homes. The purpose of the licensing act in this state (1957, replacing Code of 1954) is "to promote and encourage adequate and safe care and housing for aged, infirm and convalescent persons by both public and private agencies, by providing for the adoption and enforcement of rules, regulations and standards." The act also sets up two categories of homes to be licensed–nursing and custodial. The definition of a nursing home is what the name implies. It is a medical care facility providing qualified nursing service by licensed personnel. A custodial home (referred to elsewhere in this book as a retirement home) provides services in excess of a hotel or board and room type of operation, but not medical care.

The licensing act provided for a dual set of standards. One is for those homes that were in existence when the act was passed and another for homes coming into existence since the act was passed. The requirements for new homes, for all practical purposes, eliminated the practice of converting an existing building for this purpose.

The licensing act came at a time when there was a noticeable increase in demand for this type of facility. This has resulted in what might be called a building boom in nursing homes throughout the state. For the past six years an average of twenty-five new homes with a total of 1,000 beds have been constructed per year. This volume of construction shows every sign of continuing.

The increasing competition caused by the increase in new homes is beginning to show throughout the state. The general public is becoming more aware of nursing homes and, judging from the increasing number of complaints received, more critical. Previously, the only comparisons the general public could make were among the converted mansion types of operations. While we have many homes of this nature that provide excellent care, the general public sees only an old building that is apparently overcrowded (multiple beds in all bedrooms, dining rooms, lack of toilet and bathing facilities, etc.). Now, however, there are enough new homes throughout the state that have been constructed for this purpose that a comparison can be made to the disadvantage of the existing homes.

There has been a general upgrading of all homes within the last couple of years. Most of the administrators are making a sincere effort to maintain a good home. Unfortunately, as in all fields of endeavor, there is a certain minority that is either unable or unwilling to maintain the standards expected. It is doubly unfortunate that the actions of this minority result in the sensational magazine articles recently published that in general give the entire profession a black eye.

The availability of new beds is beginning to make the administration of the licensing act somewhat easier. At the beginning we found most of the homes were filled to capacity. It was rather difficult to attempt to enforce the licensing standards too rigidly because, as deplorable as some of the homes were, the only alternative was to put the patients into the street. Now, however, with more beds becoming available, we feel that higher standards can be expected, particularly in the areas of housekeeping and sanitation, employment of qualified nurses, and overcrowding.

It is the desire of the Department of Health to administer the licensing program on an educational rather than a strict enforcement basis. We much prefer working with a home to upgrade the quality of care on a voluntary basis, rather than dictating and enforcing standards. The majority of the homes are receptive to advice and suggestions for improving the quality of care. There are, however, a few homes where it is necessary to act as an enforcement agency. Our field staff is, at the present time, too limited to spend much time in any home. As a result, we are unable to conduct the educational program we would like and to police the marginal homes as necessary.

Index